Type 1 Diabetes
for the
Newly Diagnosed

Type 1 Diabetes
for the
Newly Diagnosed

What to Expect,
What to Do,
How to Thrive

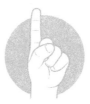

Ariel Warren, RDN, CD, CDCES

ROCKRIDGE
PRESS

For general information on our other products and services, please contact our Customer Care Department within the United States at (866) 744-2665, or outside the United States at (510) 253-0500.

Paperback ISBN: 978-1-64611-458-0 | eBook ISBN: 978-1-64611-459-7

Manufactured in the United States of America

Interior & Cover Designer: Jamison Spittler
Art Producer: Tom Hood
Editor: Lauren Ladoceour
Production Editor: Rachel Taenzler
Production Manager: Riley Hoffman

Illustration @ Shutterstock/Jamesbin, cover and p. iii
Author photo courtesy of © Alysha Kester-Terry

10 9 8 7 6 5 4 3 2 1

Contents

Introduction

This book was written to be a source of education and encouragement through your recent diagnosis of type 1 diabetes (T1D). More importantly, this book is to let you know you are not alone. You have access to communities of many potential friends who also have T1D, healthcare providers who want to help you find the right treatment based on your needs, and me, via this book, to hold your hand during the overwhelming changes that may result from a T1D diagnosis. My goal is to inspire, motivate, and teach you and your network how to better manage diabetes. Together, we can lessen each other's burdens.

Like you or your loved one, I also have T1D. I was diagnosed in 1995 when I was four years old. During that time, diabetic technology wasn't that advanced, and the prognosis didn't look great. However, being diagnosed at a young age motivated me to learn all I could about health. Doing so has allowed me to live a healthy life with diabetes and has enabled me to help many others live well with T1D.

I now practice as a registered dietitian nutritionist (RDN) and a certified diabetes care and education specialist (CDCES). I love my job as a healthcare provider because it allows me to assist people with diabetes, not only by explaining how to manage their condition, but by letting them know they are strong and capable of living a full and happy life with diabetes.

But T1D doesn't just affect the person who's been diagnosed. Parents, roommates, friends, and significant others all become part of the T1D community when someone they love is diagnosed. While writing this book, my father shared a journal entry he wrote after hearing my diagnosis for the first time. It is rather personal, but with his permission, I am including it in the hopes of providing you some comfort during this time:

This day began as any other day. It was a Thursday and Carol [Ariel's mother] and I were busy with myriad tasks: taking kids to piano, soccer, and other activities. In addition to the usual routine, Carol and I had decided that Ariel needed to see the doctor because she had suddenly started showing signs that something was very wrong.

At 4 p.m., I was at work when I received a call from Carol. She was in tears. She notified me that she was at our pediatrician's office, and he had just diagnosed Ariel with type 1 diabetes. Carol told me to meet her at the children's hospital in Dallas where they would test Ariel's blood and complete the diagnosis.

Carol arrived at the hospital with our three youngest, including Ariel, in tow. Ariel looked fine; in fact, she was running around the emergency room checking out the toys in the lobby. Once Ariel was checked in, they took us into a small emergency room where they put an intravenous needle into her right hand and a second blood sampling needle into her left hand. Ariel didn't cry when they put in the first needle, but when they put in the second, she let out a quiet sob. It's hard to describe how Carol and I felt to watch our tiny four-year-old daughter suffer.

Carol and I believe Ariel's diagnosis was triggered by a bad case of chicken pox she had six months earlier. With Ariel, the pox seemed to attack the internal organs instead of the skin. We soon found out that the targeted organ was her pancreas.

Carol and I both felt the magnitude of the diagnosis and were afraid for the life of our young daughter. Although we did not understand everything, we knew that our lives would never be the same, and that Ariel would have limitations in her life that other children would not.

Over the next two days, I stayed with Ariel at the children's hospital. During that time, I learned how to test urine, test blood, control diet, and give insulin injections. At the end of our stay, I was asked by the nurse to give my first injection to Ariel. I took that tiny needle, drew out the insulin and injected it into Ariel's leg.

I cannot describe the anguish that filled my heart as Ariel let out a small cry when the needle penetrated her skin. Nothing brought home the reality of what diabetes was more than that moment. After removing the needle and handing it to the nurse, I turned away from her and Ariel so that they would not see the tears streaming down my face. I could no longer speak. I was transfixed by the searing emotions swirling within me.

However because of great doctors, scientists, and researchers who were innovative for their time, my daughter had a treatment that allowed her to not only live, but to manage her diabetes. Through this experience, I was empowered to save my beautiful daughter, one tiny shot at a time. To me, it was a small price to pay.

. . . .

After my dad sent me that journal entry, my mom recalled a moment, "Many years after your diagnosis, you told me you were one of the luckiest people you knew. Dumbfounded by the outburst, I asked you why and you said, 'I've never broken a bone or had a bee sting!'"

I remember coming to that realization—and I still feel like the luckiest. To this day, no bee sting (although a wasp got me once) and no real broken bones (just a chipped tooth). I may have been given a heavier load than some by having diabetes but this hardship allows me to better see the goodness in life. Today, I am married to my best friend and we have two beautiful children. It may take some extra work for me to stay in good health, but I make a constant effort to appreciate the blessings I've been given.

Diabetes has taught me not to take life for granted and shown me that I am strong. Not only can I endure, I can live well through hard times. Diabetes has also given me a great level of empathy, which has allowed me to connect with others. To me, everybody has hardships— whether physical or emotional. Maybe someone has severe anxiety, depression, chronic illness, or comes from a broken home. In an odd way, beauty can spring from adversity. Hardship allows people to understand one another on a deeply personal level.

In this book, we will look at how to deal with the ups and downs of both emotions and blood sugar. We will discuss ways to find a medical team and seek out support. We will break down how to deal with the day-to-day, such as travel, work, exercise, and getting enough sleep. Finally, we will focus on how a long-term future with T1D may look. We will review the reality and possibility of reaching a more natural weight from lifestyle habits while having good blood-sugar control, being in relationships, and someday having children. The goal of this book is to give you a glimpse into what life will look like in the next few months, two years from now, and further down the line, decades after diagnosis. With diabetes, the goal is not perfection, but progression.

Each chapter starts with a real story from real people who have type 1 diabetes or have been touched by type 1 diabetes. Included in these stories, I asked my husband Jace to share one of his own personal recollections from living with me as someone with T1D (page 125). While this book is not meant to replace information you will receive from your medical provider, it is meant to fill in any holes and provide support. You will discover what works best for you, how to get through tough times, and how to rebuild so you can feel in control of your life again. As someone who also has T1D, I understand what you are going through. I'm here not only as an educator, but as a friend, to be a guide through every step of this time of self-discovery.

Sincerely,
Ariel Warren, RDN, CD, CDCES

PART I

GETTING TO KNOW TYPE 1 DIABETES

In this section, you can expect total hand-holding as we walk through the basics of T1D. Together, we will learn what T1D is (and isn't), the ways your body uses insulin and glucose (sugar), how to monitor your diabetes, and what to expect regarding life with T1D.

CHAPTER 1

THE 101 ON TYPE 1

LAUREN'S STORY

Walking into my college campus clinic, I knew something was seriously wrong. I had the classic symptoms of extreme thirst and frequently going to the bathroom, plus I was suddenly swimming in my clothes. The campus doctor suspected an eating disorder, but I threw out a guessed diagnosis: "My dad had diabetes. Can you just prick my finger so we can rule that out?"

Two hours later, I was admitted to the hospital with blood sugars in the high 500s, and a night-shift nurse handing me a syringe and insulin vial. Not a big fan of needles (who is?), I quietly cried as I pieced the sharp end into my tummy. "Phew! I did it. Never did that before," I said to the nurse. "What?! No one told me you were just diagnosed. Oh, dear. Let me give you a real tutorial."

After two weeks in the hospital with plenty more practice with injections that allowed my body to make use of the food I ate, I emerged with a fresh new 10 pounds on my frame and a bag full of insulin samples and syringes. What would come next involved telling roommates, friends, and family what had happened and that my new reality might involve a lot more planning (and pokes) than before.

What Type 1 Is + Isn't

T1D develops when someone's pancreas stops making insulin. It is an autoimmune condition that occurs when your immune system mistakenly attacks the beta cells in your pancreas. These beta cells are part of your pancreas that secrete hormones, such as insulin, which your body needs to control your blood sugar (glucose).

When you eat, carbohydrates (or carbs) break down into glucose which increases the amount of glucose in your blood. Normal functioning beta cells from the pancreas release insulin when glucose levels are too high. Once released, insulin moves the glucose from the bloodstream into your cells. Every cell needs energy (glucose), which makes insulin quite important for your body to function.

There are multiple types of diabetes. Diabetes is more of a spectrum, rather than two distinct categories. However, at diagnosis, a majority fall within either type 1 diabetes (T1D) or type 2 diabetes (T2D).

With T1D, you are dependent on insulin injections because your body either completely stopped producing—or produces very little—insulin. T2D is also known as insulin resistance. Meaning that someone with T2D usually *makes* insulin, but their body doesn't *respond* to insulin. Note that someone with T1D can also have insulin *resistance* at diagnosis or develop insulin *resistance* due to lifestyle choices.

Despite extensive research, no cure for T1D exists. However, many advancements have been made over the last century. With the combination of treatment, healthy eating, and regular exercise, you can manage your T1D and live a long, healthy, and very full life.

T1D can occur in people of any age, race, shape, or size. If you have recently been diagnosed, there is no shame in having T1D. Always remember you have a very caring community of other T1Ds, educators, and providers who are anxious to support you.

FIRST SYMPTOMS

T1D is a complex disorder. Studies have shown that T1D occurs more frequently in families who have relatives with T1D or some other autoimmune disorder. There is a 3 to 6 percent increased chance of T1D if a parent of a child has T1D. The final trigger for a T1D diagnosis is usually an environmental factor such as a virus or a stressful physiological event.

This doesn't mean that contracting chicken pox necessarily caused your T1D. People who develop T1D are likely born with a predisposition. However, there are studies working to pinpoint the exact causes of T1D to possibly delay or prevent its onset.

Common T1D symptoms include:

- Frequent urination (bedwetting in children who were previously potty-trained)
- Extreme thirst
- Extreme hunger
- Extreme fatigue
- Blurry vision
- Unexplained weight loss
- Irritability and moodiness

HOW THE BODY USES INSULIN + GLUCOSE

With T1D, your immune system mistakenly sees the beta cells in your pancreas as foreign invaders and destroys them. This process can happen over a period of weeks, months, or even years before enough beta cells have been destroyed and symptoms of T1D appear.

When you eat, your body turns carbohydrates into glucose. Glucose is the simple form of sugar used by your cells for energy. To use glucose for energy, you need insulin, a peptide hormone. A simplified way to think of this is to think of glucose as gold, cells as treasure chests, and insulin as keys. To put the gold (glucose) into the treasure chest (cell), you need a key (insulin). When all three mechanisms are available and working in balance, blood glucose (BG) levels remain in a healthy range and cells have energy.

However, with T1D, if you do not make enough insulin, your cells will not have enough glucose for energy. Once this happens, your body becomes thrifty and starts breaking down fat for energy instead. The molecules produced by breaking down fat for energy are ketones. If too many ketones are produced, you can develop diabetic ketoacidosis (DKA), a severe form of ketosis often seen upon diagnosis of T1D (see "About Ketones," page 7).

On the flip side, there are also lows that can occur if your blood glucose levels fall below target. As you are well aware, with T1D, you need to take insulin to regulate your blood-sugar levels. Relating to low blood sugar, no matter how much insulin you take, the hormone will continue its usual job of opening up cells and shuttling in glucose. The issue is that if you take *too much* insulin for the amount of glucose available, the insulin will cause too much glucose to be taken from the bloodstream into the cells, causing hypoglycemia—hypo (low), gly (glucose), emia (of the blood). Therefore, it becomes essential to monitor your blood glucose levels (see "Monitoring Blood Glucose" on page 8).

If you check your blood glucose level and it has dropped below 70, you may need to eat or drink something to bring it back up to target range. Glucose tabs are a great choice for bringing up a mild low quickly. However, if you are either not a fan or don't have access to glucose tabs, you can use other fast-acting sugar sources such as Smarties, Skittles, a mini fruit juice box, Life Savers, or a spoonful of honey.

If you have severely low blood sugar, you may feel drowsy and confused, and if left untreated, may become unconscious. At this point, blood glucose levels sink dangerously low and someone else will need to give you glucagon, a hormone that helps quickly raise BG levels. Becoming unconscious from a low is rather rare; but to stay safe, keep a diabetes medical ID on you so someone will know to call emergency services.

Keeping your blood glucose levels close to normal is necessary so you can live a long and healthy life. At times it may feel like a balancing act. Besides counting carbohydrates and giving yourself the right amount of insulin, there are other factors such as stress, illness, hormonal changes, and exercise that will also impact blood sugar. Some days, you will feel that even the breeze outside can cause a low! The takeaway is that every day you will learn something new about your diabetes. It can be frustrating too, so take a deep breath and understand that it's never about perfection—only progression.

About Ketones

Ketones are toxic acidic chemicals your body produces when it breaks down fat for energy. Depending on the person and amount of carbohydrates consumed, nutritional ketosis can be reached, which equates to increased ketone levels that don't cause harm.

It is possible for a harmless state called "nutritional ketosis" to occur when the body has access to insulin, but the insulin levels are naturally low due to low carb intake through food choices or fasting. Currently, there is no agreement on the level of safe ketones for someone who is eating this way. The conservative level is a 1.5 mmol/L threshold, but it depends on the provider.

When insulin levels are falsely low from a broken pancreas (a.k.a. diabetes), your body doesn't have access to insulin, so glucose isn't able to get into the cells and be used for energy. If insulin isn't available, glucose is bypassed and the body is forced to break down fat for energy. The breakdown of fat is what produces ketones. High ketone levels can cause the blood to become overly acidic. Left untreated, this can cause you to go into diabetes ketoacidosis (DKA) and may require a trip to the hospital.

DKA is common at diagnosis since there is little-to-no insulin by the time you are diagnosed. It is best to keep your blood sugar in check, but life happens and highs occur. Also, if you are pregnant, nursing, or sick, you have a higher chance of developing ketones at lower blood sugar numbers.

There are three main ways to test for ketones: a blood ketone meter (the most accurate), urine strips (the least expensive), and a breath ketone meter (not recommended for people with diabetes).

High ketones with high blood sugar are indicative of DKA; however, other symptoms often occur, such as:

- Extreme thirst
- Frequent urination
- Nausea and vomiting
- Fruity-scented breath
- Shortness of breath

- Weakness and fatigue

- Confusion

- Abdominal pain

DKA is usually treated in the hospital, but you can prevent getting to this point by watching for symptoms and checking for ketones when your BG is at 250 and won't come down. (For more on blood-sugar ranges, see "Normal Range versus Reality," page 8.)

Monitoring Blood Glucose

When it comes to monitoring your blood sugar, you can't manage what you can't measure. This means that by monitoring either with a blood glucose monitor or a continuous glucose monitor (CGM), you can better learn how certain activities, foods, exercise, sleep patterns, stress, and your everyday routine affect your blood sugar. The more you monitor, the more you can identify trends to know if you need dosing adjustments or if you need to change certain habits. It takes practice, but by continually monitoring, you can remain in control of your life and diabetes.

NORMAL RANGE VERSUS REALITY

When it comes to staying in control, you may wonder what exactly is "in control." Here are the American Diabetes Association (ADA) range recommendations for most non-pregnant adults:

- Pre-meal or fasting: 80 to 130 mg/dL

- Post-meal (1 to 2 hours after the start of a meal): 80 to 180 mg/dL

The ADA defines low blood sugar to be below 70, and high blood sugar to be above 180. Staying within the target range is a lot to think about, especially at first because it requires great attention to your diet, activity levels, and treatment. However, the longer you do it, the easier it becomes. Please do *not* drive yourself crazy or get discouraged when you have numbers outside these ranges. Yes, strive to reach these targets as much as you can, but when you have a high or low, treat it in a timely manner, try to learn from what happened, then move on. (For more on range variability, see chapter 7, "High-Tech Management.")

HOW TO SELF-TEST

When it comes to deciding how often and when exactly to test using a glucometer, the Standards of Medical Care recommend considering your overall needs and goals.

You'll want to have clean hands when you test; sugar on your fingers can result in a false high blood-sugar reading. A false high blood-sugar reading can cause you to dose too much insulin which would then cause hypoglycemia.

Recommended times to test more often:

- Before driving and every 2 hours during long trips
- Before, during, and after exercise
- During illness or infection every 2 to 4 hours
- During preconception, pregnancy, and breastfeeding
- Change in medication
- Use of steroids (e.g., prednisone and cortisone shots)
- If you frequently have low blood sugar
- If you are unable to notice dips in blood sugar
- If you are not achieving (your and your provider's goal) blood sugar
- During high-adrenaline activities such as parachuting or skiing

RECORDING RESULTS

With diabetes, recording data as it pertains to your blood-sugar levels, exercise routine, diet, and insulin intake can give you and your doctor the ability to identify trends and adjust as needed. With the many recording methods available, what's most important is to keep an open mind and find what works best for you. Experiment with a simple diary, use a glucometer or CGM that tracks results you can download, purchase an app, or create your own Google Doc or Excel spreadsheet. There are *many* great apps available, not only for tracking your diabetes information, but for food and nutrition, which all play a role with your management.

RESPONDING TO RESULTS

As stated previously, it's good practice to check for ketones if your levels are above 250, especially if you treated with your insulin correction dose and your blood sugar isn't coming down. Along with insulin, if you have zero patience for high blood sugar (like myself), you can also add cardio to help the insulin currently in your blood to work better so your blood sugar drops faster. It's important to note that while mild steady-state exercise such as walking is generally safe for mild ketones, you do *not* want to do vigorous exercise if ketones are present. Vigorous exercise can make ketones worse.

When you have a low, you can treat by using the 15-15 Rule: Eat about 15 grams of fast-acting carbohydrates (such as 3 to 4 glucose tabs, ½ cup of fruit juice, 15 grapes, or 1 tablespoon honey, maple syrup, or straight sugar), then wait about 15 minutes. Repeat until your blood sugar registers above 70.

Some days will feel like your blood sugar is on an epic roller coaster ride—up and down with no stops! Maybe you had a low, and the "caveman" brain turns on and all logic is out the door. Caveman brain only thinks about survival and when you are this low, caveman brain says to "EAT!" Sure, maybe you were supposed to eat just 15 grams of fast-acting carbs, but you find yourself elbow-deep into the leftover reject candy from Halloween. . . . and it's April. . . . You then, of course, have a reactive high because you ate way more than just 15 grams. Oops.

Don't worry if you seem to be having many lows, overeat, then have a crazy high. This has happened to every T1D. I remember one time in college when I ate a whole row of my roommate's funfetti birthday cake. I took responsibility, got her more cake, and we're still friends. But the point is, when the T1D caveman brain kicks in, logic takes a backseat.

After experiencing some frustrating highs and lows, stop and ask yourself, "Why did I get so low?" And then, "Why did I get so high?" Learn something new by carefully considering how your insulin dosing, activity levels, and routine may be causing the ups and downs. Make an adjustment or mental note, and move on!

DOCTOR'S OFFICE TESTS

After your diagnosis, you will meet with an endocrinologist and hear about a test called hemoglobin A1c, HbA1c, or simply A1c. The A1c test measures how much glucose over the past three months has been attached to the hemoglobin, which is the part of your red blood cells that carries oxygen to the rest of the body. The more glucose that has been attached, the higher your A1c.

Your endocrinologist (or "endo," as diabetics often call them) will use your A1c as a reference point, along with other recorded data from your CGM or glucometer to better understand how you are controlling your diabetes. The A1c result is reported as a percentage and the American Association of Clinic Endocrinologists (AACE) recommends a level of 6.5% or less (6.5% equals an average of 140 mg/dL). Research shows having a 6.5% or below greatly decreases the risk of developing diabetic complications.

Where the Type 1 Diabetic Comes In

A whirlwind of emotions often mix with confusing responsibilities that come out of a T1D diagnosis. Not to mention the fact that there's no time to settle in. Diabetes doesn't provide a "getting to know you" period; it has much more of a "code red" approach.

It's common to go through a phase of denial and guilt—if we only hadn't eaten so many cookies, if only if we had exercised more, or stressed less, we wouldn't have broken our pancreas. But remember: You didn't cause this. It was bound to come out at some point or another so don't think that if you had behaved differently you could have avoided this diagnosis from happening.

Do not think you have to solve everything today and be perfect from now on. Diabetes is a learning process and there is no such thing as perfection in management. Especially in these first days, it's about survival. Over time, you will learn how to better manage and then one day—hopefully sooner rather than later—you will feel like you have your life back. For now, be kind to yourself and allow yourself to adjust and heal.

Because I was diagnosed at such a young age, I don't remember a time when I didn't have to consider insulin at mealtimes. I can't imagine going out for lunch without scouring the menu and identifying all the carb foods, guesstimating the amount of my decided entrée, trying to time administering my insulin dose to coincide with the arrival of my food, then reexamining my food to assess if my original insulin dose was sufficient. It would be nice to just order food and eat it. However, after playing this game for so many years, I often wonder—if there were a cure and I didn't have diabetes anymore, would I miss this guessing game? Probably not.

Of course, a T1D diagnosis is bittersweet at any age. If you are diagnosed later on, you have a whole life you remember from before your pancreas decided to zonk out. During these first days with T1D, it can be emotional, scary, and a bit lonely. However, no matter what age of the diagnosis, we all have the same fundamental condition—a deadbeat pancreas.

Where Loved Ones Come In

A T1D diagnosis is a life-changing event. It's an emotional process, and it commonly causes the person with the new diagnosis to draw inward and push loved ones away. Loved ones then feel helpless because they love you and want to help but don't know how.

As humans, we all need someone who holds us accountable so we can improve. My husband is that person for me. I remember when we were engaged and I asked him to go with me to my endo appointment. As we were walking in from the parking lot, he asked what my A1c was. I replied that usually my A1c was in the 7s. Feeling a bit judged at this point, I instantly got defensive and shot back, "Below 6.5% is impossible!" He replied, while nodding his head in contemplation, "Oh, we're definitely going to reach normal levels."

However annoyed I was with his remark because I felt he didn't understand what he was asking and he was belittling all my hard work, I appreciated how confident he was. Because it's not easy or simple to go through the years with diabetes, everybody needs someone they can confide in and who makes them laugh when life begins to pick them apart. My husband is the one who listens to my complaints and frustrations, even when it's entirely self-inflicted. He's there to help keep me level-headed and maintain perspective on the important things in life.

Letting people in can be difficult, but finding someone you can talk to will help you feel validated in what you're going through—and can help you better care for yourself mentally and physically. You don't need to tell everyone and shout it from the rooftops (unless of course, that's your style), but having that special someone in whom you can confide during frustrating times can make all the difference in your health and well-being.

Frequently Asked Questions

Will I be able to eat sweets again? Yes, but eating a balanced diet with an emphasis on fiber and lean protein should be the foundation of eating for anyone—with or without diabetes. However, you can still have a treat in conjunction with a healthy diet if you take the additional insulin necessary to avoid a dramatic spike in blood sugar. Most importantly, enjoy your treat when you do decide to indulge!

I have T1D: Are my children at risk? If you have T1D, there is a slight increase in diabetes risk for your children, but not much! We will go over this topic in much greater detail in chapter 13 (see "Passing on T1D," page 138), but your chances of passing down T1D to a child is 2 to 6%. If you are worried and would feel better if you knew, you can also do a screening for your child.

How does screening for T1D work? One of the most well-known screening online networks is TrialNet. It is an international network of the world's leading T1D researchers who are finding ways to prevent, delay, and slow the progress of T1D. People are eligible for a free screening if they have relatives with T1D. During this test, five different diabetes-related autoantibodies can be detected up to 10 years before a T1D diagnosis.

Can I still have a family, career, and a full life? Yes! Many people who have grown up with T1D are able to thrive, despite the ongoing challenges that come with the disease. In an odd way, diabetes can mold you into a more responsible, empathetic, and determined individual. There is something special about people who learn to live with diabetes as they become highly skilled in their personal and professional lives. Think of diabetes not as a disability, but as an ignitor that fuels you to achieve incredible things. It's all about perspective.

WHAT'S NEXT

In the next chapter, "Understanding Insulin," we will go over this hormone in detail so you can figure out what insulin types and delivery methods work best for you. We will go over how insulin affects diet and exercise, and how to treat a high. Finally, we will break through emotional and psychological barriers relating to taking injections.

CHAPTER 2
UNDERSTANDING INSULIN

When I was diagnosed at the age of 12, over 35 years ago, I started on just one shot a day using mixed insulin types to cover my needs. Though this may not sound all that inconvenient, it didn't allow much flexibility. Later on, after having diabetes for a few years, I was switched to two shots a day and thought it was the end of the freaking world! I played sports, and thought, "How am I supposed to manage my life and take two shots a day?" Then I had an epiphany and realized it really wasn't a big deal. I adapted. I then stayed on that two-shot regimen throughout my early- and mid-20s. After college, I got married, and finally had decent insurance, so I met with an endocrinologist for the first time (up to this point, I had only been seeing a PCP). I then went to an internal medicine doctor, who got me started on an insulin pump. I went directly to a pump from the two-shot-a-day regimen. As I wore pumps for a long time, my sites would leak because of the amount of insulin I had to use, so I switched to an insulin that has double the concentration known as U200, allowing me to cut my dose in half. Using this higher concentration of insulin was a total game-changer for me! My insulin doesn't leak anymore, and I feel it works better, faster, and is much more predictable.

My point is, everyone has a treatment and insulin type that will work for them. It can take time to figure it out, but keep investigating and asking your provider for treatment methods until you find what works for you.

What to Expect

When it comes to dosing with insulin, too much and you will have a low, not enough, and you will have a high. Lows and highs left untreated can make you feel sick and keep you from being able to function like a normal human being. Throughout the years, I've come to understand that you have to control your diabetes, or your diabetes will control you.

Diabetes doesn't go away. Even when you are having a bad day, and not even on your birthday. However, diabetes teaches you to be tough and disciplined. People who go through adversities either break—or become stronger. And you, my friend, are strong.

When you are first diagnosed, your starting amount of insulin is usually calculated from your weight, ranging from 0.4 to 0.5 units/kg (1 kg equals about 2.2 lbs). If you have DKA when you are diagnosed, you may need more insulin to get you back to a normal level. After this initial dose of insulin, adjustments will be made by your provider to fine-tune your protocol. In fact, your doses are likely to change throughout your life, and that's perfectly normal. Whether someone is newly diagnosed as a child, young adult, or 50-something, chances are that everything from your metabolism, energy and activity level, stress, and diet will change simply as a result of your not being a static, fixed being. Humans change. Needing to adjust your dosage can be seen as a good thing. It means you are a living, breathing, dynamic person.

Along with everything else, you will likely need to be much more aware of how insurance plans work. One way to get a sense of your costs is to use a worksheet. Affordable Insulin Project provides a free worksheet you can access online to help calculate yearly costs (see Resources, page 159). We will cover how to choose and navigate your insurance options in chapter 5 (see "The Insurance Game," page 56).

TYPES OF INSULIN

Your provider matches the type and amount of insulin to your needs. Over time, and as new kinds of insulin become available, you may choose to try different types. If you are curious about another insulin you can ask your provider for a sample and dosing instructions. All insulins have their own onset (how quickly the insulin starts work-ing), peak (low long it takes to reach its max impact), and duration (how long the insulin lasts before it wears off). You may be given insu-lin to cover any carbs you eat during mealtimes, as well as an insulin that slowly works in the background for most of the day or more.

Categorizing short-, fast-, and rapid-acting insulins can be con-fusing. What you need to know is that regular (short-acting) and rapid-acting insulins are both considered fast-acting. The differences between the two is that regular (short-acting) has a slower onset and typically longer duration compared to rapid-acting. For T1D treat-ment, rapid-acting is usually preferred over regular (short-acting) for mealtime and correction needs. Note that in the list that follows, the generic name of the insulin is listed first followed by the brand name in parentheses.

INSULINS USED FOR MEALTIME DOSING

Rapid-Acting Insulin
Names: *Glulisine (Apidra), Lispro (Humalog), Aspart (Fiasp, NovoLog)*
Onset: *10 to 15 minutes*
Peak: *1 to 1½ hours*
Duration: *3 to 5 hours*

Regular (Short-Acting) Insulin
Names: *Insulin Regular (Humulin R and Novolin R)*
Onset: *30 minutes*
Peak: *2 to 4 hours*
Duration: *4 to 8 hours*

INSULINS USED FOR BACKGROUND DOSING

Intermediate-Acting Insulin
Names: *NPH (Humulin N, Novolin N, Lente)*
Onset: *2 to 4 hours*
Peak: *4 to 10 hours*
Duration: *10 to 18 hours*

Long-Acting Insulin

Names: *Detemir (Levemir), Glargine (Basaglar, Lantus)*
Onset: *2 to 4 hours*
Peak: *6 to 8 hours (minimal peak)*
Duration: *up to 20 to 24 hours*

Ultra Long-Acting Insulin

Name: *Glargine U-300 (Toujeo)*
Onset: *6 hours*
Peak: *no peak*
Duration: *24 to 36 hours*

Name: *Degludec U-100/U-200 (Tresiba)*
Onset: *1 hour*
Peak: *no peak*
Duration: *42 hours*

Premixed Insulin

Premixed insulin combines two different types: a rapid- or short-acting insulin to cover mealtimes, and an intermediate-acting (NPH) insulin to cover between meals. The peak, onset, and duration depend on the specific insulin types and amounts used. Examples include Humulin or Novolin 70/30, Humulin 50/50, NovoLog Mix 70/30, and Humalog Mix 75/25 or 50/50.

DOSES

With diabetes, every person is different with the dosing needed to cover their background, mealtime, and correction needs, and as people change, the dose—or setting—will also change. There are a few terms you need to know to better understand how to dose for your diabetes.

Background or Basal Insulin: Basal insulin keeps your blood sugar on target overnight, while fasting, and between meals, and usually stays consistent day-to-day. Basal generally uses 40 to 50 percent of your total daily dose (TDD). The percentage of the TDD may be increased if someone is eating a low-carb diet.

Mealtime Bolus: This bolus or dose happens before or during a meal to bring your blood glucose back to target after you eat. Carbohydrates affect your blood sugar the most, therefore this ratio lets you know how many grams of carbs are covered with 1 unit of insulin. For example, your provider might determine your unique insulin-to-carb ratio is 1 unit of insulin for every 15 grams of carbohydrates you eat.

Correction Bolus: This bolus (a.k.a. "insulin sensitivity factor or ISF") is used to bring high blood sugar back to a healthy range. This ratio lets you know how much your blood sugar will lower with 1 unit of insulin. For example, your provider might determine that 1 unit of insulin can drop your blood sugar by 50 mg/dL.

Total Daily Dose (TDD): Your TDD is simply all the rapid- or short-acting insulin you take for meals and correction plus all long-acting (or basal if you use a pump) needed in a day. This number allows a provider to calculate and fine-tune your settings, and indicates your level of insulin sensitivity or resistance.

DELIVERY SCHEDULES + METHOD

With diabetes, you may have to take insulin, but you do have options on *how* you take it.

Sliding Scale Schedule: Your dose will depend on your blood sugar just before your meal. The higher your blood sugar, the higher your dose. This method is sometimes used in hospital settings and may be recommended initially because it typically requires fewer injections—typically two to three shots total a day. However, this method has been around since the 1930s and is seen as outdated, inflexible, and ineffective for optimal control.

Multiple Dose Insulin or Multiple Daily Injections (MDI) Schedule: A type of intensive insulin therapy used to more closely mimic a normally working pancreas. The word "intensive" may sound intimidating, but think of it as more hands-on, which actually gives you more flexibility and better control. With MDI, you take a long-acting insulin to cover background needs and rapid-acting insulin to cover mealtimes and corrections. You can choose to use syringes or pens with MDI.

Syringe Delivery: Syringes are used to draw out insulin from vials. Syringes tend to be more affordable than pens and have the option of half-unit doses, but they can be less convenient than pens or pumps.

Pen Delivery: Pens are more convenient than carting around syringes and vials, because with insulin pens, the insulin comes preloaded and ready-to-go. An insulin pen is an injection device about the size and shape of a large magic marker, making it rather unassuming. However, underneath the "lid" is a cartridge of insulin. To access the insulin and dose, you simply twist a small pen needle and dial up the number of units you need to take. These small needles are prescribed with your pens.

Insulin Pump Delivery: If you are sick of injections, and want to fine-tune your treatment, consider a pump. Insulin pumps are small, computerized devices that only use rapid-acting insulin for background, mealtime, and correction needs. Insulin is delivered through a short, flexible plastic tube inserted into the fatty tissue just below the skin (like a syringe) and needs to be changed out every three days.

With your recent T1D diagnosis, you will find that sticking to a routine will make managing all the necessary blood-sugar checks and insulin injections more doable. The more you make it a routine, the easier it will be to follow, and the better you will feel. To keep it simple, let's say you are given a single daily dose of long-acting insulin and then a 1:15 insulin-to-carb ratio (CR) for meals and snacks. The following is what a typical day with diabetes may include.

6:30 a.m. You get up and take a shower, brush your teeth, and get ready for the day.

7:15 a.m. You test your blood-sugar level and are happy to see it at 126. You take an injection of 10 units of long-acting insulin for background needs plus 2 units of rapid-acting insulin to cover breakfast.

7:20 a.m. You make your usual two thin pieces of whole wheat toast plus two scrambled eggs plus ⅓ fresh avocado for around 30 grams of carbs.

7:30 a.m. You eat your breakfast along with your usual cup of coffee (including a splash of almond milk). You decide to give a little extra insulin because you've noticed the coffee, though low in carbs, seems to spike you a tad. You decide to take 1 more unit, then head out the door to work.

8:30 a.m. At school or work, you check your blood sugar and find it's at 102, but you "feel" it's dropping. A friend offers a donut, and you end up eating the whole thing.

12 p.m. Yikes! You are at 287. You guess that donut did more than you thought. You make a mental note to bring your own fast-acting snack in the future and then take 3 units of rapid-acting (2 for correction and 1 for your 14-carb lunch salad).

12:10 p.m. You eat your chicken chopped salad with blue cheese dressing and feel good about yourself because you skipped the cookies passed around by a colleague.

3 p.m. You go for a snack-size bag of popcorn from the vending machine. (*Popcorn is healthy, right?*) You didn't test this time, but you see that one bag equals about 7 grams of carbs so you figure that's not enough to worry about. You forgo the shot.

4:30 p.m. You are sitting at 183 which is higher than you'd like, but your doctor instructed not to correct unless you are above 200 as a newbie with T1D and you definitely don't want to dip as you head home, so you skip the shot.

5:30 p.m. At home, you make a beeline for last night's leftover chicken and broccoli casserole in the refrigerator.

5:45 p.m. You were so hungry, you forgot to test and take insulin. Although it's only 15 minutes after you started eating, you test and find your number to be at 222. You feel it could be worse, but take 4 units of short-acting insulin (about 1½ units for correction and about 2½ for food).

6:45 p.m. You're feeling thirsty, so you check out of curiosity. You are at 212. Annoyed that it's still up, you decide to walk the dog to help bring it down.

8 p.m. You feel a little shaky, as the walk was a little brisker than intended. You check again. Ugh. 62. A little annoyed about the yo-yo blood sugar today, but you don't mind eating a small apple since you were already feeling a bit snacky.

9:45 p.m. You are sitting around a happy 143 and wind down for bedtime.

This is just an example, but it's a realistic one. As you see, diabetes can cause quite a few adjustments to your usual schedule. Throughout it all, know that diabetes can't keep you from doing what you want and achieving your highest goals. Sure, you need to check your blood and dose your insulin, but you are just as capable, or perhaps even more capable of reaching your goals. Diabetes has a way of making people more determined, more understanding, and more of a rock star. That's you! Do not stress yourself about nailing all this down. Understand that it's a process and it takes time to find your routine.

What to Do

With insulin, there are a few things to keep in mind, starting with storage. It's best to keep unopened vials in the refrigerator and use the "first in, first out" (FIFO) rule. That way, you don't have to throw any insulin away because it's past its expiration.

Also, make sure not to overheat—or freeze—your insulin. Once, I was on vacation, and my sister, who was my roommate at the time, received a delivery of my three-month supply of insulin. For some reason, she thought I stored insulin in the freezer. When I got home to find it frozen solid, I was beside myself. Though sad to lose all that insulin, I was most concerned about how little my sister knew about what to do with it.

Insulin is finicky. If your vial or pen has been opened, it can be kept in the refrigerator or stay at room temperature. Also, insulin is light-sensitive. Pens are fine as is, but if using a vial, keep it in the box or a protective case.

When I travel, either when flying or on a road trip, I use three bags to keep my insulin cold, but not too cold: one for insulin, another filled with ice, and a third larger one to contain the two bags.

Using this method, the ice keeps the insulin cold, but because the insulin is in the box, it has no direct contact with the ice and doesn't get too cold. As soon as you make it to your final destination, transfer it to the refrigerator or keep it in a cool area.

Rapid-acting insulins go bad about a month (28 days to be exact) after the rubber stopper has been punctured. Some long-acting insulins are good for up to eight weeks, but check the manufacturer's fine print online if you are unsure.

Make sure you dispose of needles according to your local regulations. If you don't have a community program or FDA-cleared containers available, you can use a heavy-duty plastic household container that is leak-resistant, remains upright, and has a tight-fitting, puncture-resistant lid. A plastic laundry detergent container works great.

Site Management

Always inject insulin into subcutaneous tissue (the fat layer just below the skin). You do not want to inject past this layer and into the muscle because your body absorbs the insulin quicker in the muscle, so you could get a low. Good places to inject are the stomach, outer thighs, hips, buttocks, and the backs of arms because these areas tend to be fattier.

However, if you are quite lean with little you can pinch, use a short needle and inject at a 45-degree angle to keep from injecting straight into muscle.

While injecting, it's important to rotate the areas where you inject. If you repeatedly inject into the same area, your skin may become lumpy and stiff, known as "lipohypertrophy." You want to avoid this because it can lead to poor absorption of insulin and cause unpredictable highs and lows.

Personally, I always switch sides and move around in a square. For extra safety, I always check for any puffiness or irritation before deciding on my next injection site. My favorite injection sites are on my backside. The stomach is more popular, but I have never had good luck there. My advice is to find what works for you. Start with your stomach, as that's where it is FDA-approved, but then branch out as you feel more comfortable.

To avoid fat desensitizing, check for lumpy or stiff areas before you inject. It may seem contradictory, but you actually want your pump insertion site or injection to sting just a little; that usually means you aren't injecting into an affected area. If you do develop lipohypertrophy, the best treatment is to avoid the affected areas. Healing can take anywhere from a couple of weeks or months, and sometimes even up to a year depending on the severity. For clean and infection-free injections, make sure the area is clean before injecting, and never reuse syringes.

WHAT TO ASK THE DOCTOR

1. Should I never eat dessert/pizza/pasta/treats again?
2. Which insulin should I take? How much, and when?
3. What is my current A1c and where should it be?
4. How often should I test my blood sugar?
5. What is one piece of advice you wish every T1D knew?

YOU DO YOU

With all the different insulin types and treatment options, what's important is to find the right fit for YOU. Speak up to your provider if you are having trouble, closely monitor and watch for trends in your numbers, and become your own advocate.

Understand that as you change, your settings change. At times you may feel like you are a living, breathing science experiment, but every time you safely try something new or make a small adjustment with your dosing, you will discover what works and what doesn't.

Last, we T1Ds need to stick together to share our triumphs, hardships, and discoveries. Whenever you're ready, know that you can connect with other T1Ds through online communities and support groups (see Resources, page 159). By learning and sharing, we all improve our diabetes care.

Frequently Asked Questions

Will insulin make me gain weight? Without insulin, your body cannot use glucose for energy. Therefore, your body will breakdown muscles and fat instead, leading to unhealthy weight loss. Once you start insulin, you may gain weight back. Keep in mind, you may also gain unwanted water weight during this process since your body is properly processing carbohydrates once again. After you have stabilized your blood sugar along with the gain and loss of water weight, you can consider healthy weight loss with the help of a registered dietitian nutritionist (RDN) or a certified diabetes care and education specialist.

How many injections do I need a day? It depends on your choice of treatment. If you choose a sliding scale, you will use a premixed insulin consisting of intermediate- and fast-acting insulin with two injections a day. If you choose MDI, you will need a long-acting insulin and a fast-acting insulin and anywhere from 2 to 10 injections a day. If you choose an insulin pump, you only need fast-acting insulin and one infusion set change every three days.

How do I fly with syringes and insulin? You can take insulin, syringes, pens, a pump, and other supplies needed for your diabetes management on a plane. Just make sure to notify security that you have diabetes and that you have your supplies with you. Note: If you use a pump, you will likely need to be screened by TSA.

JUST ONE THING

Being diagnosed with diabetes will cause a lot of changes in your life, but some days you just need a break. Today, your mental break can be to do something NOT related to diabetes. You heard me: no diabetes. To do this safely, try keeping your carb count low so your insulin levels are also low, which greatly decreases the chances of fluctuating blood sugar. Next, think of something you loved doing before your diagnosis and have fun!

CHAPTER 3

CARB COUNTING

My husband and I were feeling adventurous, so we decided to try the all-you-can-eat sticky finger dinner at Wingers. This definitely isn't a regular occurrence, but we had been golfing all day and I was starving. I googled the carbs like I typically do. The first plate was 150 grams of carbs, including fries. I had two more plates of sticky fingers that were 40 grams of carbs each, so the whole dinner totaled a whopping 230 grams of carbs! Since I was a little low beforehand, I delayed my bolus by about 10 minutes for the first plate. I then bolused for the second plate right when I ate it but waited again to bolus for the third one until about an hour later when my continuous glucose monitor (CGM) indicated that my blood sugar was starting to increase. The next morning, I expected to wake up with sky-high levels, but much to my surprise, it never went above 120! I totally dominated that guessing game.

What to Expect

As someone with diabetes, you need to count the carbohydrates in your food to keep your blood sugar on target. Carbohydrates are one of the three main macronutrients (nutrients your body needs in large amounts) along with fat and protein. However, each person may have different requirements of the amount of macronutrients (especially carbs) needed to optimize his/her health. Some do well with higher carb, while others may do better with lower carb. All macronutrients (carbs, protein, fat) are what provide energy in the form of calories from food, with carbs being the body's primary source of energy.

There are three main types of carbs: starch, sugar, and fiber. Eating a diet high in fiber can help protect against many cancers and reduce inflammation, cholesterol, and blood-sugar levels. A high fiber diet is linked to increased insulin sensitivity, healthy immune function, and improved gut health. Fiber also promotes sustainable weight loss and maintenance. Fiber-rich foods include vegetables (especially leafy greens) and other plant sources such as beans, whole grains, fruits (especially berries and ones with a peel), nuts, and seeds.

Carbs break down into glucose and are then absorbed into the bloodstream where insulin moves the glucose into the cells to be converted into energy. Without having a fully functioning pancreas, you don't have insulin, therefore you have to be the mediator by counting the carbs in your food and calculating how much insulin you need. If you are off with your carb counts, too much or too little insulin will cause highs or lows.

Carbs lurk in many more foods than just bread and pasta. You'll find them, for example, in candies or syrups, fruits, milk, yogurt, and even vegetables (especially the starchy ones). Each of the three carb types (starch, sugar, and fiber) affects blood sugar differently and should be accounted for when counting carbs. One way to do this is to find the "total carbohydrate" number listed on the nutrition label. Then check the serving size to calculate the total amount. If you eat multiple foods, add all the carbs together from each item you eat.

If a food doesn't have a label, such as produce, you can look online to find a close estimate of carbs. One serving of fruit, starch, and milk each equals about 15 grams. Non-starchy vegetables usually contain about 5 grams or fewer of carbs per serving (about 1 cup raw or ½ cup cooked); therefore, you can eat more of them—and they are a great source of fiber, vitamins, and minerals. However, all carb sources add up. Make sure to count them all and don't be embarrassed if you need a calculator! This process may seem overwhelming at first, but we tend to be creatures of habit. Once you memorize the number of carbs in your favorite foods, carb counting becomes much easier. It's also important to be picky with your carb choices. Choose healthy, high-fiber carb sources such as berries, beans, lentils, nuts, and seeds, which are all also high in vitamins and minerals.

On the other hand, processed foods such as sugar-sweetened beverages, white bread or pasta, pastries, white rice, sugary cereals, soda, and candy are high in refined carbohydrates (such as white flour and sugar) and very low in fiber, antioxidants, vitamins, and minerals. Such foods can cause a roller coaster of highs and lows with your blood sugar and cause you to feel rather crummy.

FAT + PROTEIN CURVEBALLS

When you add protein and fat to carbohydrates, the usual carb spike is delayed and the rate of carb absorption is slowed. This delay and slowed absorption can be helpful because rapid-acting insulin takes about 15 minutes to start working, allowing the insulin to better match the speed of your rising blood sugar. This delay and slowed absorption can also keep your blood sugar from violently swinging up and down, giving you whiplash from aggravating BG swings. Bottom line: It is important to balance healthy sources of carbs, fat, and protein.

The issue comes when we get crazy and eat large volumes of all the macros. Eating foods such as pizza, alfredo pasta, cheesy enchiladas, etc. (you know, the good stuff) can cause a two-part mayhem event. First, there is the anticipated initial spike from the carbs. Then, the fat and protein kick in, which causes a second spike that is slow, steady, and extremely stubborn. This second rise typically lasts two to five hours, but can last as long as eight hours. The issue with this is that the cheesy, bready, and fatty meat food combinations are often on the menu for dinner, which can create the perfect storm for an annoying rise in blood sugar as you sleep. And when you are sleeping, you can't actively treat your blood sugar, which can cause hours of untreated hyperglycemia. Fun, right?

THE FIBER FACTOR

As I've already touched upon, fiber has many physiological health benefits, such as its potential to aid in weight loss, and its heart- and colon-protective properties, but it is particularly useful for those with diabetes because of its stabilizing effects on blood sugar. If you are not a huge vegetable fan, know that you can also find fiber in whole grains, berries, fruits with skin (e.g., pears, apples, kiwi), beans, nuts, and seeds.

The Dietary Guidelines for Americans (DGA) recommendation for adults is to eat 14 grams of dietary fiber for every 1,000 calories. This averages about 25 grams for women, and 38 grams for men per day. These amounts are the same or higher for people with diabetes. Personally, I do not go around tallying up my fiber grams for the day—that would get monotonous and it's not necessary. However, I do incorporate some type of fiber every time I eat. For example, for dinner, I make sure to take in some sort of non-starchy vegetable. If I'm eating a snack, I include another veggie or some nuts or seeds. For the great majority of people, eating fiber with every meal or snack is a sufficient way to make sure you are well above the dietary guidelines. If you are not used to fiber, *do not* go overboard all at once. You will regret it. It takes time for your body to adjust to additional fiber in your diet. Start by adding small amounts to each meal.

Being diagnosed with diabetes can trigger strong emotions—some days diabetes just stinks. You now have to examine all foods for carbohydrates like a self-scanning robot. Going to your favorite restaurant or eating at a work party necessitates more attention to detail, but it gets easier with time. When you have T1D, you become well aware (annoyingly so at times) of how much certain foods may "nuke" your blood sugar—causing it to shoot up and therefore become difficult to treat and get back to a more normal range.

Through many years of careful watching, I have found the foods that spike my blood sugar. Common foods that make the "nuke" list are those high in processed and refined carbohydrates and fat such as pizza, fries, and cereal. Although cereal is not often high in fat, it is usually high in added sugars. You will likely find that you can get away with a small amount of a nuke food, but the more you consume these foods, the more dramatic the spike, and the longer your blood sugar remains stubborn to treat. Also, there may be foods that nuke your blood sugar but don't affect someone else with T1D. Remember: These lists are highly personal, so take the time to discover what can blow your blood sugar out of whack.

What to Do

With the popularity of low-carb diets, the food industry has modified many foods to reduce carbohydrates. Unfortunately, this can make it rather confusing when you have T1D and are trying to figure out how much insulin you need to cover the turkey wrap you ate at lunch. Manufacturers have found tricky methods to get the counts down and blur the line between total carbs and net carbs.

It's important to know that dietary fiber naturally occurring from plants along with sugar alcohols may blunt, or greatly reduce, the usual spike in blood sugar. This is important because it all affects how much you will need to dose with your insulin.

It can get rather cumbersome when trying to figure the total net carbs. "Net carbs" are simply the carbs absorbed by the body that cause a rise in blood sugar. As a general (and totally optional) rule, you can subtract fiber from the total carbs if there are 5 grams or more of fiber. If there are also sugar alcohols, divide the amount of sugar alcohol by 2, then subtract that number from the total carbohydrates. Total carbohydrates – fiber (if greater than 5 grams) – (sugar alcohols ÷ 2) = net carbs.

WHEN THERE ARE NO LABELS

In today's world, we have access to nutrition labels and carb amounts at our fingertips. Oftentimes, we can search the name of a chain restaurant and entrée on our phones to get a general idea of the nutrition and carb load of a meal.

Issues arise when we are eating somewhere such as a friend's house or at an independent restaurant. This is when we need to guesstimate. Take a deep breath: It's completely doable!

First, you will need to memorize your favorite carbohydrate exchanges, which are the serving sizes of starchy foods that have about 15 grams. To get a printable, in-depth list of carbohydrate exchanges, you can use an online printable pdf provided by Lilly Diabetes (see Resources, page 159).

If you have more than 1 serving size, multiply. For example, if you ate 1 cup of rice, there are 3 servings in 1 cup. So you'd figure 3 servings x 15 grams = 45 grams.

If you eat multiple starchy foods, add them all together. For example: 1 cup of rice (45 grams) + 3 ounces chicken (0 grams) + 1 small pear (15 grams) = 60 grams.

Next, you will need to measure, which can be done by comparing the amount of starchy food with the size of your hand. One fist or cupped hand equals about 1 cup. Admittedly, this is fantastically imprecise. But with practice, eyeballing carbs will get easier and easier. For more complicated dishes, where it's difficult to account for hidden ingredients used by the chef (think sugar, syrups, reductions, heavy cream, etc.), eyeballing can be more tricky.

If I am having a really tough time guessing the carbs in a food, especially if it tastes sweet or quite rich, I will eyeball to the best of my ability, then multiply my estimated carbs by 1.25 to calculate my insulin dose. This method allows me a little extra "cushion." If it tastes too good to be true, sadly, it probably is, so give yourself a little extra insulin for better coverage. From personal experience, I have found that the extra amount of insulin is often the right amount or not enough.

If you do go out to eat, especially at a new place, it's smart to have dinner on the earlier side so you give yourself at least three hours to watch the effects on your blood sugar before going to bed. Rapid-acting insulin often used for mealtimes lasts between three and five hours in your body, with the peak of action at 60 to 90 minutes, and the bulk of the insulin used around hour three. However, the more carbs you ate, the more insulin you take, and the longer it takes for all the insulin to be absorbed.

WHAT TO ASK THE DOCTOR

1. How do I estimate my carbs when I don't know what's in my meal?
2. If a food is "sugar-free" do I have to take insulin?
3. Do I dose for net carbs or total carbs?
4. How should I adjust my insulin for protein and fat?
5. Should I change my basal, correction factor, and insulin-to-carb ratio?
6. Are there times during the day when I should have different insulin-to-carb ratios or correction factors?
7. What are some of your other patients' nuke foods?

YOU DO YOU

After diagnosis, you may have a friend or loved one question if you should be eating something. This is bound to happen, and my advice is not to worry about it. Perhaps someone finds you scarfing down a pack of Skittles, and this person can't help but ask, "Are you sure you should be eating that?" However, this person doesn't understand that you dosed too much insulin for lunch and you are now nose-diving to a low. Or maybe you just want a little piece of cake, and that's okay, too. At the end of the day, you know what is and isn't working and it is ultimately your decision on how to manage and improve your diabetes.

Frequently Asked Questions

Can I ever have delicious high-fat, high-protein, high-carb foods again? YES! However, you may feel that this triple-threat combo is a bit of work to keep your blood sugar level afterwards. A couple of tips: Try to make healthy eating the basis of your diet, but when you do indulge, enjoy a smaller portion. Also, try eating your meal earlier in the day, to give yourself time to watch and treat the induced hyperglycemia.

How do I make carb counting easier? You do not need to memorize the amount of carbs in all starchy food that has ever existed on this planet. Heavens, no. Keep it simple by sticking with your favorites and branch out from there. We tend to be creatures of habit, so although there's initially a learning curve, you will quickly learn how many carbs are in your usual meals and snacks and learn and grow over time. To help you better memorize, you can always take notes on your phone or if you keep a journal or notepad with you, record it there.

Can I eat anything I want, as long as I take my insulin? I was raised on mac and cheese, Pasta Roni, and cereal with marshmallows. My blood sugar was up and down, but I thought that was just life with diabetes. Theoretically, yes. However, you will find that your diabetes, overall health, and the quality of your life improves when you eat a healthy and wholesome diet. My advice is that it's okay to enjoy a treat here and there, but don't make treats a staple in your diet.

Take a mental break from all this tallying and enjoy a treat. Maybe you want a slice of cake at an upcoming birthday party or maybe you are traveling to Italy and are excited to eat some delicious pasta. As a registered dietitian, my advice to you is that moderation is key. Moderation is what allows healthy eating habits to stick and is a part of having a healthy relationship with food and accepting and loving your body. Personally, I love baking cookies and brownies with my son every once in a while. Do I eat the whole batch? No. But do I enjoy a square? I definitely do and I don't beat myself up about it. So today, go ahead and let yourself have a treat and enjoy it. Just make sure to take your insulin.

PART II

THE HONEYMOON PHASE

By now, you may be wondering what life will look like post-diagnosis. What can you expect, and what happens now? To help set you up for success, we'll delve into how to deal with the highs and lows, how to pick the right insurance plan and medical team, and how to cope with the emotional tolls of living with T1D.

CHAPTER 4
FLUCTUATIONS

Fluctuations will drive anyone crazy. I remember one day I was sitting in the target zone all day, so I thought, "Let's put this to the test," and I made cookies. Before I knew it, I shot up to the high 200s and it wasn't going anywhere, even after walking two miles on the treadmill. Still high, I figured the next move was to wait it out. After about two hours, my blood sugar was lowering, but at the rate of frozen molasses. Because it had been hours later, I was now hungry.

Before I knew it, I was stuffing my face with more cookies. I did a couple boluses (a bolus for each cookie and I ate three). My last bolus was supposed to be 0.7 units, BUT I accidentally bolused 7 units instead! I'm pretty sensitive to insulin, so 7 units was sure to crash me. Expecting my blood sugar to nose-dive, I was shocked to see it hardly dropped at all, maybe 20 points from 7 whole units? It just sat there in the 200s and didn't move for hours. Annoyed and tired of it all, a couple hours later it was time for bed, but suddenly, my insulin then decided to work all at once. Ugh.

What to Expect

After your diagnosis, you may wonder if you were misdiagnosed as your blood sugar may seem to be balanced with just a small dose of insulin. This phase is called the "partial remission," but is more commonly known as "the honeymoon phase." It occurs in about 60 percent of all people diagnosed with T1D. In the first year or two of administering insulin, the pancreas responds by producing its own insulin better, meaning you can greatly reduce your outside insulin doses while maintaining near-normal blood-sugar levels. This can be a source of great frustration as you deal with unexpected lows and frequent adjustments to your dosage: What worked well in the hospital may suddenly leave you crashing at home!

The duration and start of the honeymoon phase differ from person to person. However, this phase typically begins shortly after starting artificial insulin and can last weeks, months—and in some cases, even years. Because the honeymoon phase often makes diabetes easier to manage, a number of current research studies are focused on finding ways to prolong, and possibly make, the honeymoon phase a permanent period for patients.

The honeymoon phase makes management easier for a person with T1D because the remaining beta cells in the pancreas are still producing insulin. This is good news because it provides a sort of buffer against high blood sugar. Having this buffer means you do not have to be as meticulous when it comes to dosing perfectly for meals, background, and for those occasional snacks you completely forget about.

During your honeymoon phase, you may wonder if you need any insulin at all. Studies show that taking insulin can extend your honeymoon phase, but you will need to work with your provider to find the right balance for you. Too much artificial insulin will cause a low, and not enough may cause you to burn through the honeymoon phase more quickly and put you at risk for diabetic ketoacidosis (DKA). And we don't want that.

Besides taking insulin, exercise may also extend the honeymoon phase. A study conducted by the British Diabetic Association published in 2019 studied 16 men in the UK who were recently diagnosed with T1D. These men self-reported performing significant physical exercise at diagnosis and throughout their T1D follow-up appointments. These men were compared to 32 other men of the same age, gender, and body mass index (BMI) who were also recently diagnosed with T1D, but did not perform significant exercise. They measured type and duration of exercise, along with daily insulin requirement, weight, and HbA1c.

The findings of the study showed that those who exercised daily stayed in the honeymoon phase for an average of 33 months, which is five times greater than the average honeymoon phase length of only six months. This study has limitations; namely the small size, and the fact that only men were observed. However, exercise has many other health benefits, so you have nothing to lose by pulling out the rowing machine, signing up for a gym membership, or binge-watching a whole series on Netflix while running on your treadmill. No matter what you do, keeping active after a diagnosis may greatly benefit your physical and mental health *and* extend those blissful "honeymoon" days. Just closely monitor that your exercise routine isn't causing low blood sugar. If you are having trouble with lows, work with your provider to adjust your insulin dosing.

IMPROVED INSULIN PRODUCTION

New T1Ds normally enjoy the honeymoon phase, but it can also cause frustrating lows and highs. At the beginning, there may be more lows since the beta cells are still producing some insulin and artificial insulin is now in the picture and relieving some of the pressure.

At the end of the phase, your pancreas can act like a tantrum-throwing three-year-old because of how suddenly it seems to turn on and off its insulin-producing ability on a whim. This can make management a bit of a nightmare as you try to keep your blood sugar somewhat stable. When you notice an unstable trend, don't worry! Just hop on the phone with your provider to adjust your artificial insulin levels. It's a bit of a balancing act, but by working quickly and directly with your provider, you will learn how to adjust and how to treat those annoying lows and highs when they occur.

You will be scheduled to see your provider every three to six months. However, for many people with T1D, this may be their first major medical condition so you may need extra encouragement and confidence when communicating with your provider when management goes awry. Understand that getting the extra help in the beginning can pave the way for much greater adherence and success with your diabetes treatment (see more on working with your provider in chapter 5 sections, "What to Expect" and "Your Diabetes Team," pages 54 to 56).

WEIGHT CHANGE

Before diagnosis, you may have experienced significant weight loss. This happens because your body isn't able to convert glucose into energy, which forces your body to burn fat and muscle for energy instead. Without insulin, glucose from the food you eat either builds up in the bloodstream (hyperglycemia) or is excreted through the urine. High amounts of sugar in the urine will cause you to need to urinate excessively, which only intensifies the weight loss and dehydration.

Once you start insulin, your body will be able to properly utilize glucose, which is critical for your health. However, this dramatic switch can cause weight gain and rather severe water retention from your glycogen stores being refueled. This can result in around 10 to 20 pounds or more of weight gain in about a month. This is absolutely normal. Your body is just trying to stabilize itself after being starved of glucose for so long. We will discuss ways to reduce weight gain from starting insulin as well as how to lose weight in a healthy way in chapter 11 (pages 115–122).

It can all be quite overwhelming. Don't worry, my friend, the crazy fluctuations from honeymooning will get less crazy and your blood-sugar levels will become more predictable. Work with your provider, get support from your friends and family, and keep an open mind to available treatment methods. You will find your routine. Maybe you didn't get a honeymoon phase, maybe yours was short-lived, or maybe you are at the end of it and are worried about what's around the corner. If you're dealing with blood-sugar fluctuations, you are not alone—millions of people with T1D have been through this. Some days will be tough, but as long as you continue to learn, you will find methods that make management easier. It's a bad joke, but I always tell my newly diagnosed patients that now is the best time to get diabetes. Obviously, it's never a great time, but today's advancements in tech and delivery methods are amazing compared to when I was diagnosed back in 1995.

What to Do

At this point, you should be working closely with your provider as you figure out how much—and when—to take artificial insulin to achieve somewhat normalized blood-sugar levels. During crazy times of fluctuating blood sugar, I recommend moderating your carb intake. You can do this by greatly reducing (or eliminating) high-sugar and highly refined foods and sticking to a diet full of lean protein, healthy fats, and high-fiber carb sources. The best-case scenario is to avoid sugar and white flours as much as possible during your day-to-day so you can save those treats for special occasions.

I have a sweet tooth myself, but your cravings significantly decrease when you cut out the junk and focus on quality foods. If you still have a hankering for something sweet, my go-to is 70 percent dark chocolate with a handful of almonds. This treat is lower in carbs, it's creamy, has just enough sweetness, and contains healthy fat and protein, which make it satisfying. I treat myself to 1 ounce of dark chocolate and almonds after dinner.

Carbohydrates are not the enemy, although they are often villain-ized. There are many health benefits that come from fiber found in carbohydrates. However, eating too many carbs can make it tricky to manage blood sugar, especially when your blood sugar is unpredict-able. During the times of fluctuations, especially nearing the end of a honeymoon phase, your best bet is to stick to a healthy, lower-carb diet. We'll go into much greater detail about diet, how food affects blood sugar, and how to make healthy eating a habit in chapter 11.

THE END OF THE HONEYMOON PHASE

You cannot predict the exact time of expiration like a jug of milk; however, the pancreas tends to decrease its insulin production capabilities over time. Therefore, you will often see a gradual increase in insulin requirements as your pan-creas burns out. During this time, your artificial insulin needs increase, and at the tail end spatting fluctuations can occur. Think of the end of the honeymoon phase like a dimming light bulb. Over time, the filament oxidizes and becomes more and more brittle, which causes flickering during the last days of use. Then one day the bulb finally just goes out.

MAKING ADJUSTMENTS

With diabetes, expect to need adjustments. Your biggest time of change will likely be when you exit the honeymoon phase. Rest assured, life will get more predictable as you discover more about your body and how certain foods impact you. To get through this time, it is always good to work closely with your provider, but as long as you feel comfortable and you get the buy-in from your med-ical team, you can identify and make your own changes in between appointments.

Let's say your blood sugar before breakfast is usually between 100 and 150 mg/dL. You then eat your usual breakfast but find your blood sugar between 220 and 250 when you check two hours later. For the next three days, you test two hours after breakfast and find that on average your BG hovers around 180. **You found a trend.**

Since your blood sugar in our example is always above the 180 upper limit, you realize that you are likely not giving yourself enough insulin to cover your breakfast. **You found the cause.**

At this point, you decide to make a small adjustment of increasing insulin to get back to your pre-meal blood sugar within the following 2 to 3 hours. **You made a change.**

Since making the change, you continue to test before you eat, then 2 hours after you eat to see if your blood sugar has made its way back to your pre-meal number. **You monitored the change.**

Adjusting your own dosing can be intimidating—but also liberating. If you are the least bit unsure or scared, ask your provider to make the adjustments. However, you are your own best advocate, and no one knows your sleep, work, stress, exercise, and eating routine better than you do.

WHAT TO ASK THE DOCTOR

1. Do you have any thoughts on available treatments to extend the honeymoon phase?
2. How can I tell when my honeymoon phase has ended and what challenges can I expect?
3. How do I adjust insulin for highs and lows on my own?
4. Is it OK if I make adjustments to my insulin dosing on my own or should I clear them with you by phone or over email?

YOU DO YOU

Your first A1c during this phase may be surprising—perhaps higher than you expected even though you've been trying to do everything "right." The thing is, these early days are something of a roller coaster, and that's not your fault. Do not let the A1c reading at your doctor visit devastate you if it's not where you expected it to be.

Frequently Asked Questions

What is considered a small change for syringe users? If you are sensitive to insulin (your total daily dose, or TDD, of insulin is less than 40 units) increase or decrease your mealtime dose by ½ to 1 unit. If you are more resistant to insulin (if your TDD is more than 40 units), you can increase or decrease by 1 to 2 units.

What if the increased dose adjustment wasn't enough? Eat the same meal and continue with the same small increased dose for the next three days. If your blood sugar is still not coming back down to around your pre-meal blood-sugar level within two to three hours, do another increased dose adjustment. Continue to repeat this process every three days until your blood sugar comes back down to your pre-meal blood-sugar levels.

What if my blood sugar is high when I eat? If your pre-meal blood sugar is high (above 180) and you eat your usual meal and administer your usual insulin dose, but find that your blood sugar remains high, you need to remember that the insulin dose for your meal is only covering your food—and not covering the pre-meal high blood sugar. If this is the case, you can safely and easily check your correction factor. For more information, see the section titled "Doses" in chapter 2.

JUST ONE THING

Today, your mental break is to take someone you enjoy being around and go for a drive to just talk, chill, and listen to your favorite music. It may sound a little cheesy, but there is something therapeutic about driving around just to drive while spending time with someone who makes you happy. My husband and I take a random drive to nowhere often because it allows us to talk about life, our goals, and what we're excited about—all while listening to good music. Who knows, if you play your music loud enough, it may turn into a karaoke session. Which is more than okay—just let loose.

CHAPTER 5

DOCTORS + INSURANCE

I had spent several hours trying to get a supplier rep to understand how critical it was for me to have my CGM [continuous glucose monitor] right away, but my order wouldn't be available for another three weeks. I was 26 weeks pregnant and in a panic. For the most part, my blood sugar was okay, but I was constantly worried, and often just slightly over-bolusing for my needs. I was frustrated, tired, scared, and didn't know what to do.

Soon after my conversation with the supplier rep, I saw my nurse practitioner for another routine diabetes checkup. I told him what was happening, and all of a sudden, he reached for the CGM and transmitter currently in use and inserted on his arm and just ripped it off! "You are going to need an alcohol swab to wipe down my transmitter, but use mine until you get your supplies."

I can't express how much that meant to me. In order for me to use a CGM, he sacrificed his own to make sure I was safe. My point is that there are some really wonderful providers and educators out there who sincerely care about your well-being. I will always be grateful for the kindness of my nurse practitioner in that moment.

What to Expect

Choosing your diabetes medical team is one of the most important health decisions because of its great impact on your quality of life. But it can be difficult trying to find the right mix of providers you feel comfortable with and who motivate you through support, education, and encouragement.

Choosing your diabetes management clinic is a bit like dating. You don't need to commit to the first clinic you meet. You are going to visit your endocrinology clinic (a place that treats endocrine and hormonal disorders) every three to six months from now on, so definitely shop around before you decide on your diabetes team. As a side note, don't stress thinking that the clinic you choose is set in stone. If your management needs change and your clinic isn't able to help you, you can always enter back into the "dating" pool.

At the heart of each clinic is a doctor. At the endocrinology clinic where I work, the endo (endocrinologist) used to work in pediatrics, but then transitioned her practice to work with adults. With the switch, many of the patients she saw as young kids when they were first diagnosed have grown into young adults and have since sought her out again.

I see how much she cares about every one of her patients. She balances professionalism with a touch of motherly endearment, which allows her patients to accept her tough love when they need to hear it. Her patients know how much she genuinely cares, which is why they continue to come back.

Having a doctor who cares, supports, and believes in you can give you the hope and motivation you need to better manage your diabetes and be more confident in achieving your big life goals. A doctor can give you health advice all day, but you tend to listen only after you know how much your doctor cares.

Your provider is more than just a doctor; over time, he or she will come to know you as a friend rather than just a patient. Your provider will be someone who not only knows your medical history, but other personal factors such as your reactions to certain medications, your treatment preferences, your lifestyle, and who you are as a person.

When shopping around for a provider, ask yourself these questions following the appointment:

1. Did you feel your doctor was not only knowledgeable, but also clear and concise with the information given?
2. Did you feel validated with your concerns and that your questions were answered?
3. If you received less-than-optimal A1c or blood work results, was your doctor accepting? Did your doctor see this as an opportunity to discuss ways to resolve obstacles? Or did he or she use guilt or fear tactics to provoke change?
4. Were the front desk staff and medical assistant (MA) helpful and polite?
5. After your consultation, did you leave feeling optimistic about next steps to improve your diabetes and health?

YOUR DIABETES TEAM

The heart of your diabetes team will likely be a doctor or an endo, but many other key players can have great impact and even act as your main provider. Here are the professionals who may become part of your team:

Primary care doctor: A doctor, nurse practitioner, or physician assistant is the one who gives you your routine medical care, which includes physical exams, blood work, and prescriptions for medications.

Endocrinologist: Sometimes referred to as an "endo" by diabetics, this doctor specializes in diabetes and other conditions related to the endocrine system, which produces hormones such as insulin.

Ophthalmologist: This doctor diagnoses and treats conditions related to the eyes. You won't likely need to visit an ophthalmologist until about 5 years after diagnosis, but will then need to go on an annual basis to have your eyes checked for diabetes-related conditions such as retinopathy, macular edema, cataracts, and glaucoma.

Registered dietitian nutritionist: This person is an expert in nutrition. Food is a key part of your diabetes management, and a dietitian can help you learn how to eat so that you reach your diabetes, weight, medication, lifestyle, and other health-related goals (like lowering bad cholesterol or reducing blood pressure).

Certified diabetes care and education specialist: A nurse, pharmacist, or dietitian with extensive training and experience caring for and teaching people with diabetes how to go about their day-to-day routines while managing their diabetes.

Mental health professional: This person may be a psychiatrist, psychologist, or clinical social worker. These specialists can help you with mental and emotional wellness related to dealing with your daily diabetes requirements. If you feel you are showing signs of depression after your T1D diagnosis, it is important to seek help from a mental health professional. Just make sure you find one who understands the unique challenges that diabetes presents.

THE INSURANCE GAME

Working with your insurance, along with a medical supplies distributor and pharmacy, is going to feel at times like everyone is in on some big joke that you were never filled in on. If you haven't already, expect *hours* to be wasted as you are given the runaround when trying to get access to insulin (*you know*, the stuff you need to survive that should be a basic human right), along with other completely necessary diabetes equipment. However, there are ways to decrease wasted hours and make this process run much smoother:

Time your call. *Never* call on a Monday morning. You may as well waste your time watching paint dry because you will be put on hold for such a long time. Instead, check the business hours of the company or pharmacy and call during the middle of the week, 30 minutes before they close. These days and times tend to be less busy; therefore, you'll wait less.

Have a list of what you need from your doctor before calling. If the rep or tech needs something from your endo, note it and call your endo clinic ASAP. This way, you can leave a message while the information is fresh in your mind. If you're lucky, the MA will answer your call so you can get your issue resolved on the spot.

Automate your orders. When you automate, you can stock up on supplies and not have to deal with calling (and waiting) when working with a rep or tech. Just make sure you have your billing information ironed out beforehand.

> ## INSIDE TYPE 1
> It can be emotionally exhausting to handle all the details a new diagnosis brings and then determine what to do about insurance and filling prescriptions. You may find yourself extremely low on insulin yet still two weeks out before your next pickup. To help prevent this scenario, treat your second-to-last vial or insulin pen as your last. By doing this, you are never one vial or pen away from a really bad situation.
>
> If you do find yourself in a bad situation, though, call your doctor immediately, explain your predicament, and ask if they have any free samples to hold you over. If it's after business hours and your provider's clinic is closed, do not hesitate to contact urgent care or emergency services. The staff may not know your diabetes history; however, they understand that you need insulin to survive. You may get some free samples, or you may have to pay out-of-pocket for them, but again, this is an emergency at this point.

What to Do

Working with your insurance company when your preferred treatment is not on their formulary can feel like an uphill battle. Ask your provider or your provider's MA what has allowed other people with T1D to get their insurance to approve the treatment you desire. By asking those who deal with insurances all day, every day, you are bound to find a way.

We regularly help patients with this at the clinic where I work. We dive deep into any concerns, allergies, or sensitivities patients may have with their current, insurance-approved insulin (the one they don't like as much) and document these issues well. We can then take that documentation to raise a red flag and create prior-authorizations for the insulin or treatment the patient prefers and would greatly benefit from. This is just one example. My point is that if you have put in the research and have found a treatment that would benefit your health and make diabetes management easier, work with your provider and the MA to see what "magic" can be done. This may not always work, but if you are having issues with your current treatment and you and your provider feel a different route would be better for you, document all issues and complain until your insurer takes action.

HELP WITH COSTS

Managing diabetes can be expensive, therefore make sure to take advantage of the following methods to maximize savings.

Stick to the formulary: A formulary is your insurer's list of preferred medications. Sticking to this list will usually give you better coverage by your insurance.

Max out your health savings account: HSAs are only available for high deductible health plans (HDHPs), but if you do have access, max it out to pay for medical expenses. Earnings on this account are tax-free and any money not used rolls over from year to year and goes with you from job to job.

Consider gap insurance: If you can't afford your deductible, you can purchase gap health insurance which pays a fixed lump sum when you have a covered accident or critical illness.

Stay in-network: No matter which insurance plan you choose, triple check that your provider, hospital, or clinic is in-network. Oftentimes a provider will change the insurance companies with which they are credentialed, so check with your insurance to see if your provider is in-network before your visit. If not, you run the risk of having to pay out-of-pocket for the visit.

Use coupons: Ask your provider's clinic for coupon cards or any pro-grams to reduce the cost of insulin and supplies. If they do not have a physical coupon card, you can ask if they know of a coupon online. Your clinic helps people find ways to reduce treatment costs every day, so use them as a resource.

Use prescription apps: Ask your clinic if there are apps for discounts, but you can also do a quick online search for the top prescription discount results. Once you find a discount for your desired prescription, give your pharmacist the code when you order your insulin or medication.

WHAT TO ASK THE DOCTOR

1. Do you have any samples or coupon cards for my insulin and other medications?
2. If I am denied coverage, how would I go about sending an appeal to my insurance?
3. Do you have a template I can use for writing my own appeal to get a medication approved?
4. What do other T1Ds who have a similar treatment plan typically choose for insurance?
5. Do you know of a good resource to help me figure out which insurance plan would be cost-effective for my diabetes needs?

YOU DO YOU

When considering your health plan, it is important to understand your monthly premium and out-of-pocket expenses (such as copays, coinsurance, and deductibles when you undergo medical services or buy medical equipment). It is also important to look at coverage of prescription medication (such as insulin) to estimate your total costs. Understanding the insurance plans available to you and their tiers will help you better estimate expenses. If you have questions, you can always reach out to your company's human resources department. If you are obtaining insurance independently or through the government, you may qualify for savings on a plan with reduced monthly premiums and out-of-pocket costs based on your household income and size. Choosing a plan can be overwhelming, but by breaking down the key elements you can make the experience less intimidating. Remember: You can change your insurance plan every year during open enrollment. Therefore, if your treatment changes, you have the opportunity to change your plan so you receive the coverage you need.

Frequently Asked Questions

What if I am the only one in my family who needs extensive coverage?
One option is to get creative with your plans. For example, if you and your spouse are both offered insurance through your employers, your spouse could go on a low-premium individual plan, and you could go on your own HDHP plan so you only have to pay for an individual deductible rather than a family deductible.

What if I can't afford my diabetes treatment?
Check with HR from the employer who is providing insurance, and/ or the website: healthcare.gov. Through this website, you can fill out a form to see if you qualify as low-income and also be given government-sponsored insurance options. If you qualify as low-income, you can also look into programs such as Medicaid and Children's Health Insurance. Regardless of whether you qualify for low-income, let your provider know your situation. Insulin and diabetes supplies can be expensive, so it is nothing to be embarrassed about. Your provider may be able to give you free samples of medications and also let you know of available programs to help decrease treatment costs.

What process can I expect if my desired treatment isn't covered?
Ask for a prior-authorization from your provider. This may be all your insurance requires, and the MA is likely able to do this. However, if it is not enough, you will need to compile documentation and chart notes of what is wrong with your current treatment, including a letter if needed. You or the MA will submit this documentation directly to your insurance. Make sure you send it to the right contact at your insurance

company. This process may take time, but if you can get your treatment approved, it will be far less expensive than having to pay the cash price.

JUST ONE THING

Visiting your doctor can feel like you are going to the principal's office because you're worried you might "get in trouble" for lackluster blood-sugar performance. If you get in there and do your usual three-month, blood-sugar average test (which feels like getting your report card) and it's not in goal (perhaps not even close), do not beat yourself up! Diabetes can be a doozy, *especially* when you're just getting the hang of all the new changes. This is rather ironic, but after a doctor's visit, you deserve to blow off some steam by going to a favorite restaurant afterward. Of course, dose for your food and do your usual due diligence of diabetes management, but take a moment and enjoy your favorite place! And hey, you have at least another three months before your next "report card."

CHAPTER 6
EMOTIONAL TOLLS

CADEN'S STORY

Even for a headstrong, independent child like me, chronic illness is a significant burden to take on. At age 11, I managed the physical condition quite well—my parents were almost uninvolved because of how well I kept tabs on it. . . . but where I seriously suffered was in the realm of mental health. Managing a chronic condition is exhausting; the mental toll in addition to the physical toll begins to wear you out. It slowly breaks down your sense of self and identity. And like anything that is poorly maintained, there will eventually be a breakdown. Mine was in the form of an intentional overdose of insulin. Getting mental health care was the ultimate savior for me, literally and figuratively.

What to Expect

When you have a life-changing event such as a T1D diagnosis, you may experience the five stages of grief because your reality has been altered in such a drastic way. You may wonder what a T1D diagnosis has to do with grief—it's because what you're going through is considered a loss. It may not be a physical loss, but it's an emotional loss of independence and your ability to live your life on your own terms. Having lived with diabetes myself for 25-plus years, I know that while it can feel that way at first, nothing could be further from the truth. However, with a new diagnosis, you may feel overwhelmed and find yourself thinking these thoughts.

Diabetes *is* a life changer. It doesn't go away, not even during the holidays. However, by working through each of the five stages of grief—denial, anger, bargaining, depression, and finally acceptance—you will become a stronger, more determined, and more empathetic person. Life has a way of constantly putting us on an emotional path with lots of detours that try to derail us from our goals. However, as we stay committed and get through these times, we develop into people who do not take life for granted. You will ultimately learn how to fully embrace life with diabetes.

Here's a breakdown of the five stages of grief:

1. Denial: This normal reaction helps you rationalize overwhelming emotions. It is a defense mechanism to buffer the immediate shock of a loss.
2. Anger: As the numbing effects of the denial stage wear off, the pain of the loss starts to take over, which can cause you to search for someone or something to blame, to feel intense guilt, and to lash out.
3. Bargaining: This is the "what if . . ." stage—important, because it gives a temporary escape from the pain, provides hope, and gives you time to adjust to reality.
4. Depression: This type of depression is not an indicator of mental illness, but instead is an appropriate response to great loss. Common symptoms of this stage are intense sadness, decreased sleep, reduced appetite, and loss of motivation.

5. Acceptance: This refers to accepting the reality of the situation. It does *not* mean you are okay with what has happened. There's a difference.

These stages are not absolutes, nor do they usually occur in order. However, by acknowledging each stage that you are in, you can better push through until you reach acceptance. By accepting your diagnosis, you will be able to better manage your diabetes and lead a happier and more fulfilling life.

Note that acceptance is not a final state that never changes. With diabetes, you will often go through the stages in different capacities. The key is not to get stuck. The acceptance of diabetes is an ever-evolving process because you are constantly learning, experimenting, and being exposed to new research and new treatments that can positively impact your life and bring you great joy.

DEPRESSION IN DIABETES

When you have diabetes, you are up to three times more likely to develop depression. *Like you didn't have enough on your plate, right?* Depression is common with anyone with a chronic condition but it is particularly common with people with T1D because it can make them feel as if they are alone—and that no one truly understands what they are going through. Diabetes-associated stressors include:

- Feeling isolated (only 5 to 10 percent of all people with diabetes have T1D; T2D is the great majority)

- Feeling overwhelmed by everything involved with managing your diabetes

- Worrying about developing long-term complications

- A decreasing sense of control when your numbers are difficult to manage

- Feeling anxious about not hitting A1c and other diabetes-related goals

If you are depressed, talk to you doctor or ask your doctor for a referral for a trusted mental health professional. You can also make lifestyle changes to lift your spirits, such as joining a T1D support group (in-person or online), improving your diet, getting regular exercise, practicing relaxation techniques, or participating in hobbies that make you happy. You have been given a heavy load, and sometimes we need outside help to get through difficult times.

COPING

With a new T1D diagnosis you may feel a loss of control; however, there are valuable tools to help you cope. Use the following suggestions as a springboard to personalize your coping mechanisms when diabetes has you feeling overly stressed.

Breathe: As simple as this may sound, spending a few moments taking long inhalations and exhalations will help you get through the initial shock.

Get support: Reach out to loved ones with whom you feel you can be vulnerable.

Get professional education: Working with your medical team will help you with your treatment. Go to your appointments with questions and be ready to learn and grow at each visit.

Get involved: Join an T1D support group, share your thoughts, and listen to what others have to say. Aim to keep it positive.

Pamper yourself: To take care of others, you must make time to care for yourself. While managing your diabetes, carve out time to exercise, choose healthy foods, and indulge in wholesome stress-relieving activities.

When we are in a time of high stress or emotion, guess what? It affects blood sugar. Shocker. During these times, it's important to reach out to your medical team for adjustments and more education. But on your end, you can engage in certain activities to lower your insulin levels. By reducing your insulin needs, you reduce the guessing game that comes from trying to figure out the exact dose of insulin you need for food and your normal routine. A couple ways to do this is to eat a more moderated-carbohydrate diet by cutting out junk, especially highly refined carb foods, and replacing them with healthy fat, lean protein, and when you do eat carbs, choosing high-fiber sources. Regular exercise can also lower insulin resistance, but switch it up by engaging in a mix of cardio, high-intensity interval training, and weightlifting. Also, adding a source of meditation can further decrease levels while improving your mood. Enjoy some quiet time like a good soak in the tub or add a session of yoga into your weekly routine.

What to Do

Depending on your personality type, especially if you tend to be more introverted, you will likely want to close yourself off from others and "take care of everything by yourself" during your diagnosis. When you are feeling overwhelmed, it is important to reach out to others for education, guidance, and support.

During your diagnosis, your medical team should be an integral part of your support group. By opening up to your provider or diabetes educator, you can confide in those who can help you and teach you how to better manage your diabetes. If you are having trouble with nutrition, depression, or balancing life itself, communicate with your medical team so they can give you personalized suggestions.

Your friends and family can also offer tremendous support during this time. They may not have the same knowledge or education as your medical team, but they know you and can provide a safe space for you to express your feelings. It can be difficult to be vulnerable with your friends and family, but you don't have to tell everyone—just the ones with whom you interact frequently and you know can help lighten your burden.

Remember: With the Internet, you have access to a T1D community group in a matter of seconds. By positively engaging with others who have T1D, you can listen, share stories, and feel more understood by those who are in a similar situation.

REACHING OUT

Let's say you have been recently diagnosed with T1D. You have met with your medical team and you know what you should be doing; however, no matter what you do, your blood sugar won't cooperate. The worst part is, you are genuinely trying, but you have your whole life that also needs your attention. You know, the one before diabetes came along and so rudely pushed itself to the front of the line. You feel trapped, discouraged, and you don't see life getting any easier.

Take a deep breath. All this means is that you are human. Maybe you had a decent A1c, but you know that your blood sugar is rising above 300 mg/dL and crashing to the 50s throughout the week so yeah, your "average" looks good. Maybe your A1c is much higher than you and your provider want, which makes you feel like you are failing. You want to feel good. You want your life back, and preferably without the crazy mood swings.

My advice to you is always to be striving to learn and grow. Find the routine of eating, exercise, working, and socializing that works best so you can have more stable and normal blood sugar. Stick to this routine and when you are feeling good, add to it, monitor, then adjust. Repeat this process. Over time, you will find your happy place with your routine, and find how to be "spontaneous" without totally rocking the boat. Your routine may be quite limited at first, but you will learn how to have more variety with time.

1. If I am feeling overwhelmed, how do I simplify my management?
2. How do stress and high emotions affect my blood sugar?
3. Is it possible that I may have depression, and if so, what symptoms should I watch for?
4. Do you have a mental health specialist you'd recommend if I am depressed?
5. Can you connect me with a T1D support group?
6. How do I open up to my family and friends about what I am going through?

YOU DO YOU

Some days, you need to step back from it all and know: You have value. You have worth. You are enough.

Diabetes is tough. Life has a way of kicking you when you are down, but by finding joy and success through the small victories daily, you learn how to persevere even through the toughest of times. Just as blood-sugar levels are important in managing your diabetes, so are your feelings. Remember that you are not alone and that you have many people who sincerely care about you and understand what you are going through. It's okay to have bad days, but instead of closing yourself off, reach out because you have many people who want to support you when you are hurting. Be proactive and talk to friends, family, your provider, your CDCES, or a T1D community group. Share your voice and let yourself be heard so you can heal and become stronger because of it all.

Frequently Asked Questions

Why may diabetes increase likeliness of depression? With diabetes, there is the constant drill: Count your carbs, take insulin, factor in activity, stress, and consider previous reactions, monitor blood sugar, rest, eat, and repeat. . . . forever. And diabetes doesn't just affect the here and now; worrying about the possible *"what if"* long-term complications can be emotionally draining. And then there is always that one T1D you knew who was super sick or Julia Roberts in "Steel Magnolias" (*not accurate at all, by the way*). So yes, diabetes can increase the chances of depression. Diabetes takes a lot of attention, it can be so dang frustrating, and no matter how much time and energy you put into it, it never goes away. There isn't a cure, and no magical "pause" button for when you need a break. However, you *can* get ahead of it and become a better and stronger person from it all. You don't have to learn it all today. Remember, the goal is never perfection, but progression.

Do stress and emotions affect my blood sugar? Depression can greatly affect your mood and motivation, which can then impact your ability to properly manage your diabetes. With diabetes, you depend on insulin and if not used properly, insulin can cause fatality from dosing too much or too little (by accident or on purpose). Therefore, if you feel you are dealing with depression, or you have a loved one who is showing signs of depression, it is critical to get the necessary help as soon as possible. Depression also increases blood-sugar levels, making diabetes more difficult to manage. By exercising, meditating, and improving your diet, you can have better blood-sugar control and decrease depression.

What simple lifestyle change can greatly help with my diabetes and depression? A healthy diet always helps, but you may need to work with a dietitian or your provider for personalized suggestions. However, as long as you are healthy or have been cleared to exercise, leading a physically active life can be a great way to help lower insulin resistance and decrease depression.

What are symptoms of depression? With a recent diagnosis, it's normal to experience a wider range of emotions, including a period of feeling down and discouraged. Many newly diagnosed T1Ds report grieving for their past life. This grieving period is also true for the parents of a newly diagnosed T1D. However, it's important to note the difference between feeling down for a period and depression.

Symptoms that may indicate depression include not enjoying what you used to, having trouble getting things done, closing yourself off from loved ones/becoming reclusive, inability to focus, and increased alcohol or sedative use. Thoughts you may have include: "I'm worthless," "This is all my fault," "I deserve this," and "I will never be happy." These thoughts are absolutely *not* true but are signs of depression. Other signs are increased feelings of guilt, anger, irritability, sadness, indecisiveness, frustration, and disappointment. You also may experience physical changes such as: feeling very tired and sick or experiencing headaches, body pain, gastrointestinal issues, extreme weight and appetite changes, and/or changes in sleep behavior. If you have a couple of these behaviors and thoughts, reach out to your medical team as soon as possible.

If you or someone you know is suffering from depression, reach out for help as soon as possible. If you or someone you know is contemplating suicide, contact the Suicide Prevention Lifeline at (800) 273-8255.

JUST ONE THING

Take a mental break to write down a list of your hopes and dreams. It's easy to get caught up in everything that has been going on, but you are still who you were before your diagnosis. Think about the next five years and where you want to be with relationships, work, health, etc., and write it all down. Keep this special note someplace you can easily access whenever you need a pick-me-up or to remember your wonderful potential.

PART III

DAY-TO-DAY LIFE

In this part of this book we will be learning about the day-to-day that comes from a life with T1D. We talk about diabetes technology: what's available, when to consider it, and how it may make management easier. We also learn how to not only manage—but thrive—with diabetes during travel and at work and school. Finally, we examine tricks to help keep your blood sugar stable before, during, and after exercise.

CHAPTER 7
HIGH-TECH MANAGEMENT

There's always been dread when it comes to checking my blood sugar. All those pricks and pokes can be so burdensome. However, I always felt like there were roadblocks keeping me from being able to get a pump and CGM [continuous glucose monitor]. I was originally told I had to check four times a day, write out all my carbohydrates, and take classes. I was burned out and didn't want any extra work to meet any pump or CGM "prerequisites." But then, I changed endos and was asked if I wanted a pump and CGM. I asked, "What do I have to do to earn it?" My endo's reply: "Nothing." I thought she had to be messing with me, but it really was that easy. All she had to do was put in the prescriptions and in a couple of weeks I had my CGM and my little computerized pancreas (pump) delivered right to my door. After I was trained and put on my pump and CGM, it was like a breath of fresh air. Suddenly, I didn't have to have to do all the constant pricks and pokes. No more daily injections and no more blood-sugar checks! It was amazing how much stress was lifted once I made the switch to my new tech. I feel so much lighter and happier now. I'm so glad I took a chance on something new. My only regret was not switching sooner.

What to Expect

As a newly diagnosed person with T1D, you may or may not be familiar with the available tech, including insulin pumps that deliver insulin without the syringes and CGMs that track your blood sugar every few minutes without finger tests. Both come with learning curves. So if that sounds stressful, know that there's absolutely no pressure to consider switching to a pump or CGM. Less stress is always the goal when it comes to diabetes management.

You'll want to have a decent understanding of T1D (for many that's a year in) before considering a pump. Ultimately, the timing should be when YOU feel it is right. A pump removes most of the guesswork behind dosing insulin. Once your settings are fine-tuned (your provider will help you with this), all you have to do is enter your current blood sugar and the amount of carbs you will be eating. With those two pieces of data (and taking into consideration how much insulin is still working in your body—known as insulin on board or IOB), the pump makes the calculation and doses the correct amount of insulin on demand.

CGMs can be used at any point—with or without a pump. But a warning: You *will* have a love-hate relationship when you first use one. You'll love it because it'll drastically decrease the number of blood-sugar tests you have to do. The hate part comes when you have alerts waking you up in the middle of the night or during the middle of something important. For me, since making the switch, my CGM has become an indispensable part of my diabetes management and I have never looked back. Whatever you decide to do, it should be on your terms.

PUMP VERSUS INJECTIONS

An insulin pump is a computerized device that delivers only rapid-acting insulin for background (basal), mealtime, and correction needs (bolus). When considering a pump, take the time to identify your diabetes goals: A1c, time in range, and daily fluctuations with blood sugar. Think about how attaining these goals affects your life. Can you reach your goals with your current treatment or would you benefit from trying something different?

As with any change, there are pros and cons. With a pump, your expenses will be higher, and you run the risk of having mechanical malfunctions. If you have sensitive skin, you may have issues with the adhesion. You will need to change and rotate your site every three days to decrease scar tissue buildup. Also know that sites can rip off. It's not painful, but it's definitely annoying. Understand that by wearing a pump, you will have something attached to you at all times. Finally, if you disconnect the pump (on purpose or by accident), you have a higher chance of DKA.

On the bright side, pumps can be a fantastic tool to help you fine-tune your management while increasing your flexibility. You have an even better idea of how much and what is inside you since you only use one type of insulin, you can stop basal and bolus insulin at any moment, and you always know your IOB. Figure out your goals, assess if you're doing well as is or if you could benefit from either adjusting your treatment or looking into a pump. The choice is yours.

CGM VERSUS GLUCOMETER

Then there is a CGM. This small device uses a sensor that's inserted under your skin (usually on your stomach or arm) to test your BG every 5 minutes, allowing you to notice upward or downward trends in (nearly) real time. Depending on the make and model, CGMs also allow you to set multiple alerts relating to high and low glucose levels—especially helpful during bedtime.

A CGM is another device attached to you. This can be cumbersome, especially if, as with the pump, you are sensitive to adhesives. CGMs can also be costly depending on the model you choose and your insurance coverage. However, CGMs are a total game-changer in my book. Knowledge is power when it comes to being able to see how your actions affect your blood sugar in such a detailed manner. CGMs allow you to prevent highs and lows; with it, you can minimize swings while improving your A1c.

Considering a switch to high-tech management can be an emotional experience. You're trying to get your bearings, when a totally new and bizarre method is added to the mix. You may feel that the multiple dose insulin/multiple daily injections (MDI) method gives you a sense of control because you are the one injecting your insulin and know the amounts being injected. You may also have a sense of "freedom" by *not* knowing what your blood sugar is doing every five minutes (which is what you get with a CGM). If so, you're not alone. But that "freedom" comes at a cost. For example, maybe you only test before each meal and before bed, so you have no clue how drinking soda at each meal is making you skyrocket between meals. By not knowing, you could be causing harm. Using a CGM can take some getting used to, but you'll likely appreciate how useful and helpful the device can be. Either way, you are not locked in; If you try a pump and/or CGM and decide they're not for you, you can always return a pump within the first 30 days and you are under no obligation to continue to buy supplies for a CGM.

What to Do

If using MDI and a glucometer is allowing you to reach your diabetes goals and you are happy, fantastic! However, if you aren't pleased with your current management method or want to fine-tune, consider switching to high-tech management.

Start by asking your provider about available CGMs and pumps. Next, check with your insurance to make sure the recommended models are covered. This way, you don't get your heart set on one that your insurance won't help pay for. Next, do some research on your own; talk with other T1Ds (in-person or online) about what they use. Ask them what they do and do not like about their high-tech devices. Finally, gather a list of questions relating to the different pump and CGM options to ask your provider. Once you make your final decision, call your provider to move forward.

For a CGM, your provider simply writes a prescription to get you started. For a pump, you will either need to fill out a brief form (your provider will then send this to the manufacturer) or you will be given the contact information of the pump rep to place the order.

HYBRID CLOSED LOOP SYSTEM

Using a pump or CGM can make management easier and improve your A1c. But what about using both? A hybrid closed loop (HCL) insulin delivery system is not for everyone but I am a fan.

An HCL does half the work by adjusting basal every 5 minutes, working with a CGM. You do the other half by manually entering in the amount of carbs and your BG to dose for meals. The reason this is exciting is that it permits you to veer from a strict routine and allows you to eat later (or earlier) or fast entirely; exercise with fewer lows and highs; and give you controlled blood sugar readings throughout the night. An entirely closed loop system that adjusts basal and doses for meals is the goal for the future as companies continue to work to lessen the burden of diabetes.

WHAT TO ASK THE DOCTOR

1. What is the most popular insulin pump at this clinic?
2. Can you or someone in your staff train me on the pump of my choice?
3. Which CGM do you recommend for my diabetes?
4. Does this CGM have the option to easily share and download my data?
5. Are there any programs or ways to get my chosen pump and/or CGM at a discounted rate?

YOU DO YOU

In this chapter, we have covered the high-tech options available along with the pros and cons. Going high-tech can be exciting and can make it easier to manage your diabetes, but anything tech-related means there is room for technical malfunctions and concerns. Ultimately, you need to decide if high-tech is right for you; you are your own best advocate—no one better understands your routine and needs. If you do decide to go high-tech, expect a learning curve at first, but remember: "The best view comes after the hardest climb." With T1D, we are constantly experimenting with changes in diet, changes in workouts, changes in dosing, and changes in delivery and monitoring methods. When we experiment, we learn, and as we learn and keep an open mind, we get better at maximizing our health, and living a life filled with purpose and meaning.

Frequently Asked Questions

What are the components of an insulin pump? There are two types of pumps: For a tubed pump, you need a pump (of course), reservoirs, infusion sets, and possibly batteries (depending on the make and model of the pump). For a tubeless pump, you need the mini-computerized device that wirelessly connects with the pod, along with a pod pack which contains a pod and syringe to fill the pod with insulin.

What are the components of a CGM? A CGM consists of three basic parts: a sensor, a transmitter, and a wireless monitor (often known as a receiver). Many CGMs allow you to use your phone as the receiver, but make sure to check with the CGM manufacturer before getting a CGM to see if your exact make and model of phone is compatible.

What is the cost difference between pumps and MDI? It depends on the pump you choose. Tubed pumps are more expensive up front, but you still need to pay for the monthly supplies of infusion sets, reservoirs, and skin prep. Then there are tubeless pumps that cost less up front but have more expensive monthly costs. Remember, a pump and its supplies may be a pretty penny, but insurance should cover some or most, depending on your plan. A nationwide study conducted over nine years that observed people with T1D showed 4,991 people on pumps compared to 9,247 people on MDI. The total average additional cost for pump therapy compared to MDI was around $3,900 per year.

Today your mental break is to laugh. Laughing can be a great form of medicine that has a healing effect. Take a couple of minutes and search "funny type 1 diabetes meme" and click on images. Some memes are better than others, but you are bound to find a couple that make you grin, maybe even chuckle out loud. If you really enjoy one and think it can make others laugh, share it in a T1D online community group.

CHAPTER 8

TRAVEL + WORK

DAVID'S STORY

When I was about 18 years old, I traveled with my family to Hawaii for a summer vacation. Upon arriving at the airport, I realized I had forgotten my insulin back at home, cooling in my refrigerator! Thankfully, I had just put on a fresh, new pump site the night before traveling, filling up the cartridge in my pump with insulin that would last me three whole days. Because of that, I knew I would be okay until I flew from California to Hawaii, as there was no time to rush back home and get my insulin. Once we accepted the situation, my mom and I called my endocrinologist, who very kindly placed a new prescription order at a pharmacy near our hotel in Hawaii. I never fear type 1 diabetes on-the-go—if there's a will, there's definitely a way!

What to Expect

When it comes to school, work, and travel with diabetes, everything a person with a fully functioning pancreas can do, you can do! You just need to put in extra preparation and organization beforehand. When you achieve goals, you have every right to enjoy a heightened sense of satisfaction knowing you can still accomplish what you set your mind to, despite having a lazy pancreas. People everywhere with T1D are accomplishing amazing feats, and you can, too.

However, to accomplish the great—or just a normal day at the office or at school—you need to be prepared for highs and lows and sporadic stressful events. The more you know about your diabetes and how to control your blood sugar, the better equipped you'll be during such times.

Whether it's work, school, travel, or relationship-related, stress can cause your blood sugar to surge. Stress triggers an increase in the body's fight-or-flight hormone levels, as if you are being chased by a grizzly bear. The body then releases extra energy, in the form of glucose and fat. Since your pancreas doesn't properly release insulin for such situations, it causes high blood sugar that can be stubborn to treat. Here are some ways to combat this:

- Keep your carb count low (or at least moderate). By consuming fewer carbs, you can make the "guess that dose" game less dramatic. This is because guessing can create greater variability in blood sugar, which in turn makes you feel worse (and less able to perform as needed).

- Make sure you are keeping up with the basics. Not changing your site, not rotating your site, and not changing your insulin out can cause poor or unusual absorption, which can also cause unruly blood sugar.

Any time you eat, especially high-carb foods, you need insulin, and when insulin is involved, there's always the possibility of overdosing, which can result in low blood sugar. To decrease and prevent low blood sugar, closely monitor your blood sugar after meals and keep fast-acting snacks at your desk or work area, such as glucose tabs, Smarties candy rolls, regular soda, Life Savers, or some gummy bears.

Healthier options include raisins, applesauce cups, small juice boxes, grapes, or a small apple or orange.

Ideally, you want pure glucose or simple carbs because simple carbs without protein, fiber, and fat will raise your blood sugar the fastest. The quicker you can raise your blood sugar, the better, as that means you'll get back to your normal, functioning self quicker. A small protein snack may be useful if you find yourself with persistently low blood sugar. A few great protein-packed options are peanut butter, hard-boiled eggs, cheese sticks, or some nuts and seeds (although you might not be super popular if you snack on hard-boiled eggs at your cubicle).

From personal experience, I suggest steering clear of candies you really like, or you will find it tempting to eat when you aren't low blood sugar—especially if you tend to snack out of boredom or stress.

TRAVEL + VACATION

Traveling can be stressful. You have to pack everything (clothes, toiletries, electronics, wallet, your ID, perhaps your passport), arrange for someone to drop you off and pick you up at the airport, and arrive with plenty of time to get through security and board the plane without running like a crazy person out of fear of missing your flight. You get it. On top of everything else, you have to pack all your diabetes supplies, make sure you have a backup plan if something goes wrong, manage blood sugar (especially accounting for travel-induced stress), and get through security all in one piece.

Thousands of people with T1D have traveled and you are going to be just fine. You just need to know what to expect and how to be prepared. As you are well aware, you now need insulin and various sharp objects to manage your diabetes: lancets for testing, syringes or pens for giving insulin. Which is where you and TSA may have to communicate so you are on the same page.

Diabetes-related supplies such as insulin, syringes or pens, lancets, glucometers, pump supplies, you name it, are all allowed through the checkpoint once they have been screened. To make things go more smoothly, separate your diabetes equipment from other belongings and include a note from your doctor. Before the equipment goes through the screening machine, let the TSA guard know that you have diabetes. He or she will then nod (because this is a very common situation) and continue with the usual screen unphased.

Every once in a while, something odd will happen. Perhaps you experience a dramatic change in time zones . . . maybe you are stuck sitting for 10-plus hours because you are traveling across the world . . . maybe your insulin vial or pen is ruined, and you are out of insulin. Although any of these situations may be frightening in the moment, remember that people with T1D live everywhere.

WORK + SCHOOL

With all that comes along with balancing work or school life *and* T1D, you don't need to walk around with a name tag that says, "Hi, I have diabetes." However, I recommend you share with at least one person whom you consider a friend. That way, if someone finds you pale and nearly passed out at your desk, there will be at least one person who knows it's not because you had a wild night at the pub, and will act fast to grab you a juice rather than a coffee. In such moments, you need someone to act quickly, so it is best to have at least one person who knows your condition.

Personally, I don't make a habit of word-vomiting that I have diabetes without an intro or context. However, I'm not shy if it comes up organically in conversation. Also, at school and work, I feel safer letting more people know I have diabetes because then I have a much better chance of getting the help I need if I ever find myself in a predicament.

If you are a student and attending school away from home, you have a lot on your plate. As a T1D in college, you will experience lifetime memories and friendships just like your peers. However, by having T1D, you have added pressures, such as taking exams while your blood sugar is yo-yo-ing, drawing attention to yourself for eating snacks in a "no-food" zone, or getting called out because your professor thought you were pulling out a phone, instead of your pump.

This happened to me once in high school. I was looking at my pump for some reason and the substitute teacher asked me to bring her my "phone." Being a smart aleck, I shortly replied, "I can't. It's attached." She thought I was trying to be cute, so she persisted, but this time without any humor in her tone, "Bring me your phone, now!" I replied, "It's literally attached, it's my pancreas." I then lifted my tubed pump in the air and tugged on it. As soon as she understood what I said, her cheeks turned bright red. Looking back, I should have talked to her in private and been more respectful, but in the moment, I felt the opportunity was just too good to pass up.

Awkward situations can arise any time someone doesn't understand— or is unfamiliar with— something. That something just may be your diabetes. When this interaction occurs, take it as an opportunity to find the humor in it because life is much better when you can laugh instead of get offended. People are curious, and a great majority are helpful and kind and want you to be safe. You don't need to tell everyone, but tell those who you think should know, and tell enough people so you feel safe.

INSIDE TYPE 1

School and work can be intimidating with a new T1D diagnosis, but by eating lower-carb meals during times of stress, keeping convenience healthy snacks and glucose tabs on hand, and monitoring your blood sugar closely, you should be more than capable of managing with school, work, and while traveling.

However, your first time going back to work or school post-diagnosis, may make you feel anxious, and this is completely normal. If you get nervous, remember that people with T1D work, go to school, and travel all the time without a blink-of-an-eye! You just need to talk to your provider beforehand, and ask for a diabetes preparation checklist, then find your routine. If something goes wrong, learn from the experience so you can prevent it from happening again in the future.

What to Do

Before traveling or simply leaving home for school or work, you need to be prepared. Create a checklist of your usual supplies, figure out how long you will be gone, and bring double the supplies you'd normally need for that time frame. If you are on a pump, bring your backup plan, such as a vial or pen of long-acting insulin with syringes or pen needles in case you have a pump malfunction.

Even if you are careful, highs and lows will happen. Maybe you forgot to take your long-acting insulin. Maybe you have a bad pump site or perhaps you are stressed out of your mind because of finals or a big presentation. For this reason, I keep snacks and glucose tabs available. It's also important to eat when you are hungry (or if you are low). If you are feeling fine, and you are not in charge of your schedule, you can extend your usual non-eating times until you are hungry. However, if you go longer than usual between meals, make sure to monitor your blood sugar more closely to avoid a low.

TRAVEL TIPS

Traveling may cause you a little anxiety, but after a couple of trips and bringing the right supplies, you'll find a routine that works for you.

- Make copies of your prescription, emergency contact info, and travel letter, and stash in a variety of bags (carry-on, checked baggage, purse, etc.). Make sure your prescriptions are for generic names to reduce confusion if you need supplies from a pharmacy in a foreign country.

- Attain a backup glucometer and test strips (ask your provider).

- Figure out how many days you will be traveling, then double the supplies you would usually use for that number of days and include a glucagon nasal spray or kit in case of severe hyperglycemia.

- Keep fast-acting energy sources (such as glucose tabs and raisins) on hand in case of lows.

- Learn key words relating to diabetes if you are traveling to a place with another language.

1. Can I get the following information printed?

    - A medical note to share with travel security and my work so I can carry my insulin, diabetes supplies, and glucagon.
    - A list of my current prescriptions, including the generic names.
    - My current pump or MDI management and backup plan settings.

2. Do you have an extra glucometer I can have for my backup plan?
3. Can you review my sick day plan with me? *Ask specifically about what you should do if you become too sick to eat or drink including how much background and mealtime insulin you would need to keep safe.*
4. Can you show me how to use glucagon in case of an emergency?

YOU DO YOU

When it comes to travel, food is a part of the full cultural experience. By embracing another culture's food, we can learn about those from another heritage. In this case, I would say to go ahead and try the food you are unsure about but use your best guess with the carbs. One approach is to fill a quarter of your plate with the unknown food and fill the rest with foods you recognize and know the carb counts. Such a method will allow you to have a deeper cultural experience without throwing your diabetes completely out of whack.

Frequently Asked Questions

What about TSA screening before I fly? As your first time flying with diabetes, it is completely normal to feel a bit anxious. However, TSA screens people with diabetes who carry their diabetes supplies every single day. Though this procedure may be new to you, it is nothing out of the ordinary for the TSA staff. That said, if you have any questions prior to traveling, you are more than welcome to call the TSA helpline toll-free at 855-787-2227 or visit the TSA website: www.tsa.gov.

What if I'm low and I don't have fast-acting sugar foods? Fortunately, candy, fruit juice, soda, or fruit are usually accessible almost everywhere you go. Go to any convenience shop or food stand and stock up so you don't run into this situation again. Skip candy that contains chocolate, nuts, or caramel because they contain protein and fat which can delay your blood sugar from rising as quickly.

What are healthy convenience foods for travel? For health reasons, I enjoy mostly plant-based and low-carb snacks such as nuts, seeds, nut butter packs (such as peanut or almond butter), hard-boiled eggs, ready-made chia seed packs, carrots and peanut butter, avocados, roasted edamame, and fresh berries.

How do I discreetly take a shot or test? Lancing your finger or taking out a syringe and injecting can make you feel uncomfortable the first few times, but don't let your discomfort stop you from taking your insulin. You need it to live! However, if you feel uncomfortable doing so in a public setting, seek out a private, well-lit location. Bathrooms are not ideal due to sanitary concerns, but you can look for out-of-the-way places such as an unused office or a low-traffic area. If it makes you feel better, I have never had an odd reaction, but then again, I'm not waving a flag and using a mic to draw a crowd.

For a mental break, take a moment to choose one place you want to travel, and fantasize about going there within the next three years. The only catch is that it needs to be somewhere that takes at least five hours of driving or two hours of flying to reach your destination. The purpose of this goal is to have you branch out of your comfort zone and encourage you to continue to travel and explore as a healthy T1D who can do anything a non-T1D can do.

CHAPTER 9
BEING ACTIVE

JESSICA'S STORY

I have always been someone who likes to stay fit, and I decided not to let diabetes stand in my way. I love to ski (both water- and snow-) and lift weights. I have run a couple of Ragnar races, and I like to trail run. I am not superfast, nor do I even work out every day, but I know how to manage my blood sugars to allow for exercise to be a part of my life. If I want to try something new, I try it. Most recently, Stand-Up Paddle boarding (SUP) in the mangrove fields in Cancun. Life with diabetes is still my life, the life I want to lead, with an extra facet of adventure thrown in. I can do anything anyone else can do!

What to Expect

Exercise can be a great tool for managing diabetes. It may require a bit of experimentation to discover how different types affect your blood sugar. But once you do, you can unlock benefits for your overall health, mood, and body composition, and ward off long-term complications.

With exercise, there are two main categories: oxygen-rich aerobic (running, biking, walking, swimming, and dancing) and oxygen-restricted anaerobic (heavyweight training, sprinting, or any exercise that uses short and intense exertion). It's important to distinguish between the different types because the intensity and breathing dictate what mechanisms your body uses for energy—which then affects your blood sugar.

Aerobic activity, especially after about 15 minutes or more, will lower your blood sugar due to enhanced insulin sensitivity and increased glucose uptake by the contracting muscles. However, if you took too much insulin before an aerobic workout, the enhanced insulin and accelerated glucose consumption by your muscles will cause your blood sugar to drop. If you didn't adjust your insulin before your aerobic workout, you may find yourself inhaling glucose tabs like there's no tomorrow.

On the flip side, you can expect a rather different reaction from an anaerobic workout. With this type of workout, you may see that your blood sugar dramatically spikes, and then is followed by a delayed drop. Don't worry, this is completely normal. It's merely a surge of stress hormones—a.k.a. an "adrenaline rush"—which increases the demand for energy (glucose) needed by your muscles. These stress hormones reduce the usual effectiveness of insulin, causing it not to work as well initially. Once your muscles have sent out the distress call asking for more energy, your liver responds by dumping stored glucose into the blood. The issue is if you do not have enough insulin available, especially since the insulin is not working as well, the rise in glucose from your liver cannot get to the demanding muscles. You will then see a spike in blood sugar. The more exertion, the more stress hormones released, the less effective your insulin, combined with the increased demand for glucose from your muscles—the higher the spike in your blood glucose levels. To add to it, the more intense and prolonged the workout, the longer and greater the enhancement with insulin sensitivity later on. Enhanced sensitivity is a good thing, as long as you know how to adjust for it. If you don't, you may experience persistent lows for hours after your workout.

Such factors are why many with T1D have the misconception that they cannot exercise. All the "rules" of exercising with diabetes can make someone with T1D feel it's not worth it, but when you find how to make exercise work for you, it is absolutely liberating. It becomes an exciting tool for better management.

BENEFITS OF EXERCISE FOR T1D

I see exercise as my secret weapon. I work out six or seven times a week but I vary my intensity and keep it fun. If I find my insulin needs increasing, I buckle down and add in more high-intensity workouts. If I experience high blood sugar after a meal, oftentimes I'll walk on the treadmill or break out the mop and polish the floors for a good 15-minute cardio session. If I wake up and my morning fasting blood sugar is a little on the low side, I bust out sprints on the treadmill. Those are killer, but they definitely cause a rise in my blood sugar and are effective for muscle toning.

How I see it is that diabetes is a fantastic motivator to keep up your exercise routine because of how it can help lower insulin needs. Once you understand how different types of exercise affect you, you can use exercise to improve your diabetes and get all the other associated cardiovascular, mood, stress-reducing, and weight-maintenance perks that go along with it.

DURATION + INTENSITY

Knowing how the different types of exercise affect your blood sugar will open a world of better workouts and more stable diabetes control. However, first make sure you have been cleared by your doctor for activity, especially if you have any conditions that would make exercise a threat to your health.

After you know you are clear, start slow and increase the duration and intensity over time. The American Diabetes Association recommends 150 minutes of moderate-intensity exercise per week. When you break it up, that's 30 minutes, five times a week (with no more than 2 days between). If 30 minutes is too much for you to do at once, break it up into 10-minute chunks throughout the day. Also, to get the full benefits you need to stay consistent, space out your workouts, and perform a mix of aerobic and anaerobic workouts. Staying consistent means to continue to exercise. Getting in a great workout is awesome, but likely not going to happen every time. Staying consistent is about continuing to work out, even if it's super short, or not all that intense. A good routine to use is two to three sessions of weightlifting with a mix of two to three cardio sessions throughout the week.

What to Do

I work out fasted (meaning before my first meal of the day) for two reasons. First, without food in my system, I have lower insulin on board (IOB; just background); therefore, I do not have to worry about my blood sugar nose-diving from the insulin becoming more effective during the workout, especially if it's cardio-based. Second, working out on an empty stomach makes for a more effective session for accessing fat to be burned because glucose from a recent meal isn't available. As a side note, I always drink water during any fasting, which is especially important for those with diabetes in order to keep kidneys, liver, brain, and digestion healthy.

The only time I run or do cardio after I have eaten food recently is if my blood sugar is hovering higher than my target, or I see it is going up. To me, it's exciting and fun to be able manipulate exercise for my advantage. Here are a few different scenarios of how I use my blood glucose numbers to determine the type and intensity of my workout:

Fasting blood glucose between 80 and 130: If I wake up here, I don't eat, and I am free to do whatever type of workout I choose.

Fasting blood glucose between 130 and 200: Above 130 before a fasted workout and I begin to feel nervous. For my management, I would then make half my usual correction and then stick to 2 to 3 miles of steady-state, moderate-intensity cardio. The cardio will initially cause a mini spike of about 10 to 20 points in BG, but then after about 15 minutes, my blood sugar will start to lower.

Fasting blood glucose below 80: Do *not* exercise when your blood sugar is this low. Stop your workout and eat some glucose. However, if you are in a workout and above 80 but trailing down, you can add in anaerobic exercise or sprints to make your blood sugar temporarily spike. This spike in glucose takes at least 5 minutes to occur after the anaerobic exercise, therefore you will need to do this early-on before your blood sugar hits 80.

Note: Intense anaerobic activity can initially spike blood sugar but will then cause you to have lower blood sugar later in the day due to increased insulin sensitivity.

Fed-state blood glucose between 140 and 250: When this is the case, I'll set out to run/brisk walk for 15 minutes to get my insulin moving to more quickly bring down my blood sugar. However, I do not exercise, especially vigorous exercise, if ketones are present (see chapter 1, "About Ketones," page 7). The recommendation to check for ketones is if your BG is 250 mg/dL or higher.

If you are able to, my advice is to work out fasted and base the type of workout according to your blood sugar. Working out fasted greatly reduces lows; this means that instead of having to pop glucose tabs mid-workout, you'll get a great session in (without having to add in additional calories). If you can't workout fasted maybe because of certain medications or a hectic schedule—between family life, work, and running errands—reduce insulin levels beforehand. To do this, either work out 2.5-plus hours after a meal (especially if that meal was higher in carbs), or if you are working out soon after a meal, keep the meal lower carb. No matter what, it's about consistency in the number and types of workouts. It does not have to be a killer workout every time. Shoot, some days the only way I can get myself on the treadmill is by watching Netflix on my phone as I go. What matters is to do want you can, try to find enjoyment, and stay consistent.

MONITORING BLOOD SUGAR

If not managed properly, exercise of any kind can cause scary lows. This is not meant to discourage you from being active, but to let you know how crucial it is to monitor and test before, during, immediately after, and then once an hour for a few hours after exercise.

Low blood sugar occurs most often within the first 45 minutes of starting aerobic activity. The risk of hypoglycemia is highest for at least 24 hours after an intense workout, and the greatest risk of nocturnal hypoglycemia happens from working out in the afternoon. Here are some strategies to decrease exercise-induced hypoglycemia:

- Avoid injecting insulin in the muscle that you will be using. Doing so can accelerate insulin absorption and cause hypoglycemia.

- The "golden zone" for before, during, and after exercise is 100 to 180.

- If you're below 90 before a workout, eat or drink 5 to 20 grams of fast-acting carbs.

- Prioritize aerobic over anaerobic exercise if you are between 181 and 270.

- If above 250, check for ketones before exercise (see chapter 1, "About Ketones," page 7).

- Take notes. Jot down what happened when you lifted weights, versus when you walked or ran three miles.

- Have fun! Be proud of what you accomplish.

Figuring out how you respond to exercise takes time. Every person is different and needs an individualized plan. Be patient, start small, take notes, and make sure to pack some fast-acting sugar in case of a low.

WHAT TO ASK THE DOCTOR

1. How often should I check during the night after a workout?
2. What should be my blood-sugar target before bed after an intense workout?
3. Do you recommend a bedtime snack after a workout done in the afternoon or later in the day to avoid nocturnal hypoglycemia?
4. How should I dose for the meal following a workout?
5. Should I adjust my long-acting insulin for a workout?
6. Do you have any available resources or referrals to help me learn how to exercise with T1D?

YOU DO YOU

Generally speaking, aerobic activity (cardio) brings your blood sugar down after about 15 minutes. This drop increases the longer you exercise and the more insulin you have onboard. The high intensity of an anaerobic workout tends to cause a spike in blood sugar, then a delayed drop, and then increased insulin sensitivity for hours afterward. A mix of the two tends to keep your blood sugar more stable during your workout, but also causes increased insulin sensitivity afterward.

By using these rules, you can develop your own workout routine that's best for you. If you put in the effort, you can become a master of exercise for better control. Yes, it can be frustrating, but is it also so rewarding when you get it right. The key is not to give up, and when you have a low or an annoying high, own it, learn from it, and keep trying.

Frequently Asked Questions

What is a good exercise routine? A mix of aerobic (cardio) and anaerobic (high intensity resistance training) is ideal for reducing insulin levels—meaning two to three sessions of cardio and two to three sessions of resistance per week. You can also mix your cardio and resistance by doing a training session that uses aerobic and anaerobic exercises. For example, you could do a steady-state run with intermissions of weightlifting, burpees, squat jumps, push-ups, or other heart-pumping movements.

How do I keep my reduced insulin needs consistent? My advice is to spread your workout days throughout the week. For example, if you are starting with three workouts per week, don't bunch them up over a three-day period; instead, space them out. For optimal results, don't go longer than two days between workouts.

What if I don't have time to exercise? You can get in a killer HIIT (high intensity interval training) workout in just 10 minutes. Everyone has 10 minutes. These types of workouts tend to be more anaerobic based, so watch for a spike and treat accordingly, but research shows that HIIT workouts are quite effective for increasing insulin sensitivity and for fat loss. There are many free workout videos online so you can do it from anywhere. If you only have 5 minutes, create your own workout and keep it simple. An example workout would be jump squats, mountain climbers, and burpees for the finisher!

For your mental break, put your knowledge into practice. Tomorrow morning, do something active before you've eaten breakfast. That could be dancing to your favorite songs, taking a long walk, or going to the gym. For example, if you are mildly above target, preform steady-state cardio. If you are in range, do a mixed workout. If you are a bit on the lower side, start with anaerobic activity, then switch to mixed. Closely monitor how your blood sugar is affected (especially if using a continuous glucose monitor [CGM]). Don't worry if you have an unexpected reaction, it takes time to craft the skill.

CHAPTER 10

SLEEP

Going low in the night has always been a cause for concern for me; however, I didn't realize the effect lack of sleep had on my diabetes. Sleep used to be my favorite thing. That all changed when I became a mom. I haven't gotten a full eight hours of sleep in nearly two years. During this time, my blood sugars have been all over the place. It's hard to make changes to my basal rates because every day is a different challenge. Last night is the perfect example of the impact poor sleep has on managing diabetes. My son currently has hand, foot, and mouth disease. Last night, he went to bed at 7. By 9, he had woken up twice, and my blood sugar was 112 and stable. He was awake from 11 until 4 a.m., then he woke up two hours later for the day. By then, my blood sugar was 256 and rising. Did I eat after 9 p.m.? No. Was there a kink or knot in my pump tubing? No. The high was simply from getting around two hours of sleep. The rest of the day I made correction after correction. Needless to say, sleep is no longer my favorite thing. In fact, it's my biggest source of stress. It also plays a major role in how my day (and my blood sugars) will go.

What to Expect

There's no denying it. Having to get up to test your blood in the middle of the night because of diabetes isn't a part of anyone's ideal sleep routine. Let's say you have a fun late night and order pizza. Sure, it was delicious, but now it's 1 a.m. and you are dealing with a low from being overzealous with the insulin at first, then around 4 a.m. you have a high from not having enough insulin to cover the spike from all that delicious high-fat cheese. Those with T1D just can't seem to catch a break! If it's not pizza, it's something else. Maybe you had an amazing intense workout in the late afternoon, maybe you ate out with some friends and had a little wine, maybe your in-laws are coming over and they send your cortisol levels through the roof. Life happens and it affects your blood sugar even while you sleep.

Interrupted sleep is the norm for those with T1D, but that doesn't mean that it doesn't negatively impact your health and well-being like everybody else. An article published by *The Wall Street Journal* reported that interrupted sleep may be even more detrimental to overall mood and thinking ability (like memory and focus) than having less sleep. The reason is related to how suddenly we are jerked out of deep sleep, which decreases our time in deep sleep, which affects glucose metabolism and hormone secretion which is what can affect blood sugar. Ah! So yes, sleep affects diabetes. Shocker. Deep sleep is when your energy and cells regenerate, which allow your muscles to better heal (especially after a tough workout), and for tissue and bone to repair. Deep sleep also strengthens your immune system. Unfortunately, as T1Ds, we have to contend with both: no sleep and interrupted sleep.

HOW SLEEP IMPACTS DIABETES

Poor sleep negatively impacts how your body responds to glucose. Even a single night of bad sleep can decrease insulin sensitivity by 14 to 21 percent. This can make for a bad day of trying to figure out the right insulin doses for meals, correction, and background. If bad sleep becomes a habit, your insulin resistance can rise, which also increases your risks for microvascular (retinopathy, nephropathy, neuropathy) and macrovascular (coronary artery disease, peripheral artery disease, and stroke) diabetes-related complications and weight gain.

Recommendations for sleep from the American Academy of Sleep Medicine (AASM) to promote optimal health suggest children (ages 6 to 12) should sleep 9 to 12 hours, adolescents (ages 13 to 18) should sleep 8 to 10 hours, and adults should sleep 7-plus hours. Unfortunately, the majority of people do not meet these criteria, and the numbers are even smaller for those with T1D.

Another factor relating to poor sleep is sleep variability, or day-to-day changes in bedtime and sleep duration. High sleep variability often occurs with teenagers, but can happen to anyone who doesn't keep to a regular sleep pattern. For example, this happens when someone stays up late and sleeps in on the weekend, but then has to wake up early for work or school during the week. High sleep variability affects your body's circadian rhythm, which is your internal clock that responds to natural daylight and darkness. High sleep variability not only increases insulin resistance, but also makes it more challenging to keep from eating and grazing on poor food choices. This behavior can contribute to weight gain and make it harder to manage blood sugar.

HOW DIABETES IMPACTS SLEEP

Studies show that people of all ages with T1D experience lighter sleep and less deep sleep compared to people who are of good health and without diabetes. And among people with TID, those who sleep more than six and a half hours per night had a lower A1c compared to those who sleep less than six and a half hours per night. (Remember, the ideal range is 6.5% A1c or lower.)

Clearly, sleep and diabetes can either be a vicious or a virtuous cycle because the two greatly impact each other. When you get at least seven hours of uninterrupted sleep on a regular schedule, your insulin levels decrease and your blood sugar is more predictable and easier to manage. Sleep has also been found to help you achieve a healthy weight, improve your immune system, lower your risk for heart disease and other metabolic issues, and improve mood and productivity. However, as you know, poor sleep has negative consequences. Poor sleep increases insulin needs and can cause more erratic blood-sugar levels. Other health issues from poor sleep include an increased risk for dementia, depression, mood swings, and certain cancers, while increasing the hunger hormone called ghrelin, which makes us more snacky for sweet, salty, and starchy foods.

Diabetes doesn't hit pause when you go to sleep, which can make it rather difficult to get a restful night. Nighttime highs are frustrating because you are unable to correct so you stay elevated for hours which then can increase your A1c and the risk of developing complications. On the other hand, lows can be scary especially if you are unable to feel the lows (known as hypoglycemia unawareness). If you are newly diagnosed, you will likely be able to feel your lows and wake up to treat them, thus avoiding a severe low that could otherwise turn into a diabetic seizure. So yes, lows can be scary, but by adjusting insulin and medications, your exercise timing, and watching your alcohol intake, you can decrease your night-time hypoglycemic risk.

Also, devices such as a continuous glucose monitor (CGM) combined with an integrated insulin pump can either stop or adjust your basal to prevent lows. If you decide against the fancy pump, a CGM by itself can alert you so you can treat with a fast-acting carbohydrate before a severe low occurs.

What to Do

A good way to prevent nighttime low blood sugar is by controlling your blood sugar throughout the day. Doing so allows for more pre-dictable blood sugar so that lows are milder and easier to prevent. If you are bouncing from high to low all day, you will likely have to give larger doses of insulin to bring your blood sugar down. The larger the dose, the greater the chance the amount is too high, the higher the chance of a severe low. Also, reducing carbs (at least before bedtime) and monitoring your blood sugar more carefully will also decrease the risk of you having a scary low during the night. Otherwise, there are some general things you can do to help improve sleep:

- Aim to keep your blood glucose under control during the night (80 to 140 is ideal)

- Make sure your room is cool, well-ventilated, and dark.

- Make sure your room is noise-free or try a noise machine to drown out disruptive noise.

- Stick to a regular sleep pattern and schedule.

- Avoid drinking fluid two hours before bed.

- Avoid caffeine a minimum of six hours before bed.

TREATING NOCTURNAL LOWS

How I explain symptoms of severe low blood sugar is that when you get that low, your brain is lacking glucose and you are not working on all cylinders. At this point "caveman brain" turns on and all logic is out the window. Once caveman brain takes over, the only thought going through your head is: "FOOD IS SURVIVAL!" You may have been given the 15-15 rule, which is to eat 15 grams of fast-acting carbohydrates, then wait 15 minutes to see what happens with your blood sugar. Yeah, no. That's solid in theory and works well, but completely irrelevant once caveman brain has been activated.

So what happens when caveman brain causes you to chug an entire bottle of juice and down a bowl of Lucky Charms with extra marshmallows? By the time you get a sense of the grand total of carbs you just inhaled (usually after about 15 minutes), your BG is already well on its way to skyrocketing to the moon. The level at which caveman brain is activated differs from person to person. To avoid activating caveman brain at night while you are trying to sleep, explore the following:

1. If you are using a CGM, set a low alarm a little above where you usually start to feel low. A good number to use is 80.

2. Keep your fast-acting snack choices to 10 to 15 grams of carbs (such as 3 to 4 glucose tabs, ⅓ to ½ cup of fruit juice, ½ cup regular

soda, 10 to 15 Skittles or grapes, or 1 tablespoon of honey, maple syrup, or straight sugar).

3. Use fast-acting food that you don't particularly enjoy to decrease the likelihood of binging. Keep a stash in your nightstand.

4. If you have been having persistent lows, it is good practice to eat a protein food *after* you have given your body 15 minutes to absorb the fast-acting carb. Nuts and seeds are great options for protein-rich foods that can easily be stashed in a small baggie in your nightstand.

WHAT TO ASK THE DOCTOR

1. Should I adjust my blood-sugar target while I sleep so the alarms don't wake me up as often?
2. How do I limit necessary blood-sugar checks during the night?
3. How can I increase my detection of low blood sugar if I am starting to experience hypoglycemia unawareness?
4. Within what range should I aim to keep my blood sugar during the night?
5. What types of snacks are good to eat if I am having reoccurring lows?
6. How quickly is it safe to go back to bed after treating nocturnal hypoglycemia?
7. How do I safely adjust my insulin dosing if I am having reoccurring nocturnal hypoglycemia?

YOU DO YOU

The markers for good sleep are to have enough hours for your age (7+ for adults, 8 to 10 for teenagers, 9 to 12 for kids), to go to bed and wake up around the same times each day, and to sleep without disrupters. Then of course, the last marker is to keep your blood sugar within the golden zone of 80 and 140 throughout the night.

Let's pause and be realistic. The golden zone takes work to accomplish and sometimes it's simply not going to happen. If you are setting your nighttime goal to be within this range but it's interrupting your sleep because of a blaring CGM alarm or continual blood-sugar check, you may need to relax your nighttime target range for a bit, as long as you stay safe, so you can have better sleep.

Frequently Asked Questions

What can cause an urgent low blood sugar? When glucose in your bloodstream isn't balanced with the insulin present, high or low blood sugar occurs. Too much insulin in relation to what you need causes hypoglycemia, possibly urgent hypoglycemia. So, too, does skipping a meal or engaging in vigorous exercise (without adjusting insulin) as well as certain medications, dose changes, or the type of insulin. For instance, NPH should be considered carefully since it is known to peak in effectiveness four to eight hours after injection (see "Types of Insulin," page 18). Taking NPH before bed can thus cause an urgent low during the middle of the night.

What is considered low and urgent low blood sugar? A blood sugar below 70 is consider low and can be harmful to you, but a blood sugar at or below 54 is considered an urgent low and requires immediate action. The lower your blood sugar is and the longer it stays low, the higher the risk for a severe hypoglycemic episode (experiencing unconsciousness or a diabetic seizure).

What do I do if I fear low blood sugar, especially during the night? Fear of hypoglycemia (FOH), especially during the night often leads to ongoing high blood sugar. Constant elevated blood sugar can be harmful to your body and will increase chances of diabetes-related complications. However, treatments such as cognitive interventions (focusing on changing thoughts) along with relaxation training can be used to decrease anxiety caused by low blood sugar. Lastly, consider a CGM. By using a CGM you can sleep, assured that you'll be alerted if you do go low.

What are ways I can decrease uncontrolled blood sugar during the night? The best way to keep your blood sugar stable is to go to bed with low levels of insulin and active carbs on board. You can do this by eating a lower carb dinner that's chock-full of filling vegetables, lean protein, and some satisfying fat. However, if you do need to treat a low, eat just enough to treat and keep it to fast-acting carbohydrates.

JUST ONE THING

For a fun mental break, take a few minutes to shop online for an item that could improve your sleep. For example, if your bedroom isn't dark enough, consider switching to blackout drapes or investing in a nice sleep mask. If your bedroom is too hot or stuffy, consider looking into an air purifier that is also a fan. Research reviews to find a product that's within your price range, then make your purchase. If you didn't get a good night's sleep and it's affecting your sugars the next day, remember that you always have another night ahead to reset and get the rest you need.

PART IV

THINKING ABOUT THE FUTURE

By now, you may be wondering how T1D will affect your long-term future and life plans. Having a chronic condition definitely impacts your day-to-day no matter your age, but it doesn't have to limit your dreams. Still, it's good to have an idea of what adults living with T1D experience and how they manage some of the more, well, adult parts of life.

CHAPTER 11
WEIGHT GAIN + LOSS

JOSH'S STORY

Shortly after returning from our honeymoon, I told my wife that I felt like I was in a diabetes rut and needed to have a complete overhaul to once again be the standout patient I had been as a child. With her support and my doctor's empathetic attitude, I made my desired changes and saw immediate improvements. I felt better, my numbers were more consistently in range, I was working toward transitioning to a CGM [continuous glucose monitor], and I was . . .

Fatter? How could that be? With astounding speed, I noticed my body changing and swelling. Within four months I went from a springy 165 to a bulging 205 pounds. I scheduled a meeting with my doctor. What I learned was that a prolonged period of poor blood sugar management had led to my body being perpetually dehydrated and starved. More than a few of my consumed carbohydrates were never being metabolized as my kidneys frantically offloaded the excess. When suddenly my body had the proper amount of insulin, my body was free to store up all that glucose. My dehydrated cells and intercellular space swelled with the osmotic changes to my blood, and boom, 40 pounds were born.

What to Expect

It happens: the freshman 15, holiday parties, or simply losing sight of eating a balanced diet. At some point in many adults' lives, they find themselves wanting to lose weight. Losing weight can be difficult, but when you throw in a chronic condition that affects hormone levels, all craziness breaks lose!

There's no sugar-coating it: Weight loss is tough. Weight loss with T1D is tougher, but not impossible. Let's say you decide to change up your diet by adding more vegetables instead of dismissing them as you previously had. Perhaps you are not necessarily changing what you are eating, but the amount. Now instead of using the mixing bowl for cereal, you are going with an actual cereal bowl. Perhaps you are jumping all in and changing what you are eating *and* the portion sizes. This leads us to where T1D and weight loss don't exactly see eye-to-eye. With diabetes, you will likely be on a fixed dosing schedule and when you reduce or change what you eat, you increase the chances of having a low because the previously dosing worked just fine and now it is too much. And then of course, how do you treat a low? Food. But not just food, straight sugar, which isn't exactly on anyone's weight-loss friendly foods list.

Then you need to factor in exercise, which affects blood sugar in all sorts of wacky ways. Typically, steady-state cardio or moderate-intensity exercise lowers blood sugar; mixed usually keeps it somewhat steady, but then reduces it later on; and then high-intensity exercise tends to spike it—then lower it—and can sometimes cause it to be lowered for up to 24 hours (see chapter 9). And yet again, we are having to treat with more sugar. *Awesome.*

Of course, treating lows is one thing, but when you keep getting low and say, "To heck with it all," and instead of grabbing the small mini juice box, you grab the whole dang gallon and gulp it down until you "feel" good, you invite trouble. An hour later, you'll likely be sitting at 300-plus. Which then means you have to take more insulin. However, when insulin levels are too high for your maintenance needs, the insulin causes your body to store the extra energy as fat for later use. This means insulin levels that are too high can make weight loss difficult.

Now that I've officially bummed you out, understand that there *are* ways to lose weight with T1D. It may take some time to dial it all in, but once you learn how exercise affects blood sugar, how to adjust insulin dosing to avoid lows, and how to improve the nutrients and quality of your food, you can shift to lifestyle habits that allow for weight loss that sticks. Don't get discouraged when you get a low, or an occasional reactive high. It happens to us all, and you are more than capable of losing weight in a healthy and sustainable way with T1D.

INSULIN + WEIGHT GAIN

At any given moment, your body is burning glucose for fuel—unless you are eating a strict low-carb diet. If your fuel (glucose) is more than the amount of energy being burned, your body will convert the excess into glycogen (very compact glucose) and store it in your muscle and liver. In between meals, when your glucose levels drop, your body breaks down the stored glycogen into glucose for energy. This is a very normal process. However, when there is excessive glucose available and the muscles and liver have met their glycogen fills, the body is forced to store it as fat.

Think of glycogen as the food in your refrigerator (skeletal muscles and liver). It is easy to get food out of your refrigerator, but there is limited storage there. Think of body fat as frozen food in a giant freezer (fat cells) in the garage. This food in the freezer is much more difficult to get to and the food inside the freezer takes longer to prepare; however, an abundance of frozen food is available in the freezer. This body fat (freezer food) is used when insulin levels are low due to unavailable glucose (fresh food) or glycogen refrigerator food.

Without insulin, your skeletal muscle, liver, and fat cells are cut off from glucose which then causes the breakdown of fat and muscle for energy and artificial weight loss to occur. The insulin is the missing key, and now there are dangerously high levels of blood glucose and acidic ketones. When your blood glucose levels become too high, some of the glucose passes into the urine and you essentially "pee away" the food you ate. These events can exacerbate artificial weight loss because of the unnatural loss of water and energy (glucose).

There is a healthy—and a harmful—way to lose weight. Unfortunately, women with T1D are 2.5 times more likely to develop an eating disorder. An eating disorder is an illness that occurs when someone experiences severe disturbances in their eating behavior, thoughts, and emotions. People with an eating disorder typically become consumed by thoughts surrounding food and their weight. There are three main types of eating disorders for the general public: anorexia, bulimia, and binge eating disorder. However, people who have T1D have an additional eating disorder known as diabulimia.

Diabulimia is a type of bulimia unique to T1D where someone will purposely skip or reduce their insulin in an effort to lose weight. Skipping the insulin is seen as the "purging act" which is how diabulimia was coined. Diabulimia is a very serious condition. If left untreated, it can lead to severe DKA and cause coma or death.

Due to the seriousness of diabulimia complications and associated increased mortality risk, it is critical for one who may have diabulimia to not delay getting professional help. If you think you may have diabulimia or any eating disorder, make sure to contact your endo to ask for his/her recommended referral so you can get the help you need.

What to Do

It can take your body as long as a year to truly stabilize after diagnosis, and perhaps even longer depending on the severity of your diagnosis. It's important to understand that this is a time of healing; it's not a time to beat yourself up about weight fluctuations that are out of your control. However, you can achieve good health and weight through healthy lifestyle choices after diagnosis and in the far future should weight gain become an issue after the honeymoon phase has passed.

Changes in weight can be rather emotional, especially if you are blindsided and are sensitive about your weight (and really, most people are on some level). When you first start insulin, a large portion of the rapid weight gain is related to your body resetting its vastly depleted glycogen storages. Each gram of glycogen stores 3 to 4 grams of water. When glycogen stores are completely depleted this can result in around 10 pounds or more of "water weight" loss.

Therefore, when insulin is started, your muscles and liver are going to have a heyday replenishing their utterly drained storages. However, additional water weight is also common as your body is trying to adapt to being able to use insulin again. This can make you feel rather "puffy," but understand that this is completely normal, and your body will adjust to a more natural state now that you're giving it insulin again. Take this time to allow your body to restore health, and get back to feeling good and vibrant again.

SAFE WEIGHT LOSS

Using insulin as you should will not make you gain extra weight but will restore your body to the natural weight that you should be based on your lifestyle choices. However, high levels of insulin for anybody (with or without diabetes) can impede weight loss goals. Strategies to lower insulin while maintaining healthy blood sugar:

Avoid hypoglycemia: Not only does low blood sugar cause you to eat more than you would otherwise, it also means you are using too much insulin. Too much insulin promotes an increase in fat stores and weight gain.

Moderate carbs: Eating too many carbohydrates, especially from refined and highly processed foods, can significantly increase required insulin dosing. Make the basis of your diet full of lower-carb, high-fiber foods such as non-starchy vegetables, and balance with protein and healthy fat. Eating this way will allow for a reduced total daily dose (TDD) of insulin.

Avoid nuke foods: These foods are commonly high-carb refined foods, but it's different from person to person. What makes them "nuclear" is that they cause your blood sugar to spike and be unresponsive to your usual correction dose. To decrease TDD, keep such foods to a minimum.

Exercise regularly: Having regular sessions of both cardio and high intensity or resistance is effective for increasing insulin sensitivity. The more sensitive you are to insulin, the less insulin you need overall.

Know your insulin: Certain basal insulins have a higher risk of causing low blood sugar (NPH is one, because it peaks four to eight hours after injection). Using an ultra-long-lasting insulin that has a minimal peak (if any) decreases the chances of low blood sugar. A pump, especially an integrated hybrid closed loop pump that continually adjusts your basal, may further decrease insulin needs because it eliminates unnecessary insulin doses.

WHAT TO ASK THE DOCTOR

1. How can I limit weight gain from taking insulin?
2. How do I lower my TDD of insulin while keeping healthy blood sugars?
3. What type of diet should I eat to reduce insulin needs?
4. What type(s) of exercise are best for losing weight?
5. Is there a particular sustainable weight loss method you have seen to be most effective?
6. How do I know if I have an eating disorder?
7. If I were to change one thing in my care for healthy weight loss, what would be your recommendation?

YOU DO YOU

By exercising, eating a majority of whole foods that are moderate in carbs, yet balanced with protein and fat, and by dosing adequately for your needs, you can lose weight while keeping your blood sugar in control.

Some days you may not feel as motivated, other days you may have a low (or a couple) and have to eat fast-acting sugar. But it's okay! This is a learning process. To get started, don't overwhelm yourself with a bunch of changes, start with just one or two changes in the way you eat and exercise. Next, set each goal while considering the following:

What: *The behavior you want to change.*
How often: *The frequency you will do this.*
Be realistic: *The goal that's achievable for you now.*

For example: *"I will eat a handful of nuts (**what**) instead of a piece of candy five days out of the week (**how often** and **realistic**)."*

Understand that every effort gets you closer to your goal, even if the effort is just learning "what not to do." Be patient and be realistic. Sustainable healthy weight loss takes time.

Frequently Asked Questions

How do I lose weight when I have to treat for lows? One way to do this is to keep a "carb reserve" for lows. Meaning that if your goal is to eat a certain number of carbs per day (which greatly varies depending on your approach), leave about 15 grams for treating lows. If you end up low, you can treat without exceeding your "budget."

What foods should I be eating for weight loss? The vast majority of those who do not have a chronic health condition would benefit from a diet that: is high in non-starchy vegetables (such as broccoli, kale, and leafy greens); meets the minimum protein (animal or plant-based) requirements (0.8 grams per kilogram of body weight); and includes fat with an emphasis on plant-based sources such as avocados, nuts, and seeds. Keep to foods that have few ingredients on the label, or better yet, foods that don't require a label, such as fresh fruit (especially berries) and vegetables, nuts, and seeds.

What are signs of diabulimia? The first and most common sign of diabulimia is weight loss without trying. Other signs include: feeling very thirsty and tired; thinking or talking a lot about body weight and image; mood swings or depression; hiding blood-sugar records with A1c readings; being secretive about food, insulin, blood sugar, or eating habits; canceling doctor appointments; eating more often (especially sugary foods); fruity breath (sign of ketosis); high stress; hair loss; dry skin; and excessive exercising. If you or a loved one show these signs, seek professional help today or tomorrow. Diabulimia is a serious medical condition that can be fatal.

JUST ONE THING

For your mental break, head to your kitchen and grab a large trash bag. Today you are going to "declutter" your life of foods keeping you from reaching your health goals (regardless of whether you're trying to lose weight). Any type of decluttering, especially relating to food, creates a sense of confidence and self-efficacy. Grab a bag and toss all foods that are not good for your health or diabetes (candy, chips, soda, etc.). Only exception is to keep what you use to treat a low. Get rid of everything else—and ASAP so it's not sitting around to tempt you. If some items may be beneficial to someone else, you can donate them.

CHAPTER 12
RELATIONSHIPS

One morning, I woke up to find my wife unconscious. Immediately, my adrenaline kicked in and I started running around our apartment in search of any sugar. I ripped open a bag of candy and started to force-feed her. However, it was too late, and she wasn't cognitive enough to chew. At this point my panic went into full gear.

Out of desperation and fear of losing her, I sprinted toward the nearest store. In my haste, I had left barefoot in the dead of winter in Utah. When I got to the store, my heart dropped because there was a huge line. On the verge of tears, I announced: "My wife is in a diabetic coma, and I need to buy some orange juice. NOW!" A moment later, with juice in hand, I sprinted back to my wife.

Once I got back to her, I started pouring the orange juice down her throat and waited for her to react. My mind started catching up with the reality of what had just happened, and I broke down and wept. But then, I started to hear little crinkles of candy wrappers and little faint giggles. She was coming back! I can't explain the relief that swept over me.

For the next while, we just sat there, holding each other. I was determined to never let this happen again.

What to Expect

Managing T1D can be overwhelming. On top of having to closely monitor your blood sugar, find the right treatment, and take care of your mental health, you have to consider how it all affects your relationships.

As humans, relationships with others are vital for our emotional and mental well-being. A healthy relationship is when any two people love, support, and encourage each other, functionally as well as emotionally. In a healthy relationship, you should not only feel safe with that person, but you should motivate each other to pursue your dreams and be able to share commonalities with your life goals. A healthy relationship is built on mutual respect, trust, honesty, good communication, problem-solving, being understanding of each other's needs and differences, and knowing how and when to compromise when you don't agree.

All relationships (including romantic, work, friendships, and family) need to be maintained and require effort to grow. In a relationship regarding a significant other, it's common for your significant other to worry about you because they care and don't want you to get hurt or sick. Oftentimes when a significant other gets upset, it comes from a place of worry because of how much they care. Although every relationship has its own set of challenges, having a healthy relationship as the foundation can allow diabetes to be something that unites rather than pulls you apart.

Common stressors for your significant other regarding your diabetes include uncontrolled blood sugar that increases the risk of severe complications. Your significant other will likely want to help you deal with your daily diabetes routine as it may affect other responsibilities such as taking care of the family, running errands, and engaging in your professional work life. Your significant other may also want to know what to do if there is a diabetes emergency. Diabetes can also cause a sizeable toll on your finances with all the necessary doctor visits, medications, insulin, and supplies. Diabetes can be frustrating and overwhelming and can cause you and your significant other to experience a lot of emotions. However, having a partner you can count on and who is understanding and empathetic can go a long way toward making the experience less stressful.

By opening up and being vulnerable, both of you can talk about how your diagnosis has impacted each other's lives. This conversation will allow you to brainstorm how to help each other during certain scenarios such as being prepared for spontaneous outings, establishing healthy boundaries during periods of high or low blood sugar, and knowing when to call emergency services during severe circumstances. By openly communicating, you will likely learn how your significant other feels, why they get upset at times, and how much they truly care. Such a conversation will also help your significant other better understand why you may say hurtful things during times of low blood sugar and why you get so irritable during times of high blood sugar. By being able to confess, talk about, and then brainstorm your diabetes-related or any general concerns, you will be able to draw closer to and relay on each other during times that call for more emotional and physical attention.

MOOD SWINGS

Diabetes can affect much more than blood sugar. When you are battling highs and lows, intense mood swings will likely occur and cause you to say or do things that can be hurtful to those closest to you.

As a finely tuned organ, your brain needs to use one-half of all the sugar in your body due to the density of neurons. However, if someone is eating a very low-carb diet, the brain can access glucose through gluconeogenesis by using glycerol (the backbone of fatty acids) from ketones. The problem is that when there isn't enough glucose (because you are experiencing a low), neurotransmitters (the brain's chemical messengers) are not produced and communications between neurons break down. Because of this, low glucose levels can lead to loss of energy for brain function which is linked to poor attention, decreased cognitive function, and sometimes changes in mood and behavior.

If you say or do something that is uncharacteristic of you because of uncontrolled blood sugar, understand that this is normal behavior given the circumstances. However, you can limit these mood swings by more closely monitoring your blood sugar and thus preventing the high or low from ever occurring. If testing your blood sugar with a glucometer isn't enough, consider using a continuous glucose monitor (CGM).

Friends and family may struggle to understand mood swings brought on by uncontrolled blood sugar; however, educating them on why high or low blood sugar occurs, how it makes you feel, and how they can help you during an episode, can help them better understand you—and strengthen your relationship at the same time.

DATING + SEX

Diabetes can make putting yourself out there difficult, but there is a certain someone looking for you, and all the qualities that have made you into who you are, which includes diabetes. When it comes to dating, there is no need to rush into spilling your guts about the woes of having a chronic autoimmune condition. It's not exactly light and fuzzy conversation material.

However, by keeping it light, perhaps even throwing diabetes out as a joke, you can get it off your chest but in a way that's not a total mood killer. For instance, my go-to during my dating days during college was, "My pancreas decided to quit working, so I had upgrade to this shiny tiny robotic one instead." At which point, I'd pull out my insulin pump. Then without another word, I'd put in back in my pocket and not say anything else about it. By not saying anything else, it dramatized the moment, but still kept it unserious. This method made for a lot of good laughs.

I'd say a good majority of your date prospects will not know very much about T1D (we are bit of a rare kind). If they do "know," they may say something offensive like "Oh yeah! My grandma got that from eating too many treats, but she just takes pills." Don't worry, your date didn't know better, but you are definitely welcome to walk out of the restaurant on the spot. By bringing up your diabetes, you will be able to weed out the good eggs from the bad. The good will be sympathetic, yet curious, about you and what makes you who you are.

When it comes to intimacy, lots of things can impact your desire. Maybe you have a fear of going low, maybe you are irritable because of a high. Whatever the fear or reason may be, the more you communicate about what you are experiencing, the better your partner will be able to understand and help.

Sometimes problems are not related to your current blood sugar but to sex itself. Common for men with T1D are erectile dysfunction or problems ejaculating. While, women with T1D may experience problems with arousal, vaginal dryness, and discomfort from sex relating to the vaginal dryness.

If you are suffering from sexual dysfunction, instead of closing yourself off from your significant other, try to communicate what is wrong. Most common dysfunctions can be treated. However, by not communicating, your lack of intimacy and silence can make your partner feel undesired—which can hurt your relationship.

INSIDE TYPE 1

To have a healthy relationship, you have to communicate. Period. To communicate, you must express yourself, talk about your ideals, your big goals, your fears, and who you are as a person.

Talking about your diabetes can make you feel vulnerable because it is something that you cannot always control. But guess what? As humans, we *all* have things we can't always control and we *all* benefit from having someone else we can talk to when times get tough. We all have our "stuff." Diabetes is your "stuff." By having diabetes, you have a deeper empathy for those who have not had it easy. This common ground allows us to understand one another, regardless of the cause of the hardship.

What to Do

The quality of the relationship with your significant other impacts your overall health and diabetes control. A healthy relationship is when two whole people with separate lives come together to share their lives. They have their independence, their healthy boundaries, yet they are there for each other to be supportive and helpful during difficult times. Having a healthy relationship allows you to better manage your health, diabetes, and better cope when times get tough.

On the other hand, studies show that a relationship high in contention and stress can negatively affect your heart, immune system, and blood sugar. Relationships, however good or bad, can greatly impact your general well-being and diabetes.

You can improve your health and your relationship at the same time with the following suggestions:

Learn together: Have your partner go to your doctor or CDCES visit(s) with you. Having your partner come along will make you feel more supported and your partner will be able to better understand what you need from him or her to improve your health.

Share goals: Improved nutrition and exercise goals can be priorities for everyone regardless of having diabetes. By setting and sharing goals together, you can increase accountability and build each other up, which yields a greater success rate.

Nurture the relationship: Set aside time to spend time doing something fun to bond as a couple and to get a mental break from it all.

Be grateful: Gratitude has been shown to increase empathy and protect from stress. Feeling thankful for the people in your life not only helps boost a sense of belonging, but increases your happiness within all of your relationships.

Seek help: If you need help, there is no shame in seeking out a couple's therapist. Often, a few sessions from an impartial observer can help you illuminate the issues, allow you to get it out, then address them.

For men or women:

1. How can I reduce mood swings when I have uncontrolled blood sugar?
2. What are symptoms of sexual and bladder problems?
3. What is the association of depression and sexual problems?

For men:

1. Can I test my testosterone levels?
2. What treatments are available for low testosterone and what are their side effects?
3. What treatments are available for erectile dysfunction and ejaculation problems?

For women:

1. What fertility problems may occur because of diabetes?
2. How do I treat and reduce yeast and bladder infections?
3. What treatments are available for poor arousal, vaginal dryness, or loss of feeling during sex?

YOU DO YOU

By talking with your significant other, you can express what level of their help is needed when you experience high or low blood sugar. That way, they will be able to support you without causing both of you to get up in arms. This is especially helpful when you are unable to help yourself. Also, by having "rules" before highs or lows occur can help treatment go much smoother. For example, a rule could be that if your significant other feels you are acting loopy, he or she can ask you to test your blood without you snapping back. However, he or she cannot abuse this and pester you to test at other times when you are not acting low.

Also, warning your significant other that you will likely say or do something that is hurtful during a diabetes-induced mood swing will allow them to safeguard themselves beforehand. I hate to say it, but trust me, this will happen. Feelings will get hurt, but as you communicate and learn from your experiences, you will find the right amount of help and support needed, and during a BG swing, your significant other will learn how not to take unkind words too seriously.

Frequently Asked Questions

How can I improve my relationship with my significant other? Diabetes is stressful, not only on you, but on your significant other. It's one thing to have to deal with diabetes firsthand, but to have to watch your loved one struggle with something that has serious consequences if it isn't properly managed can be quite difficult for your significant other to witness. However, by making time for each other so you can talk about your frustrations and what is and isn't working, you can help your partner understand what you are going through and how they can better help you. Also, being honest and talking face-to-face during these deep conversations allows you to approach the discussion with the attention and focus it deserves. During these talks it can be easy to get defensive, but by trying to read intentions rather than dissecting each word said, you will better understand the true aim of your significant other. Plan at least one date a month to spend time together doing something fun that gives you a mental break from it all. You can keep it as simple as going out to your favorite restaurant, just make sure to keep to that once-a-month routine.

How can I treat (or prevent) sexual problems? Monitor not only your blood sugar, but also your blood pressure and cholesterol levels. Also, achieving a healthy weight, quitting smoking, and being physically active can help with sexual dysfunction. Finally, if you think you may be suffering from depression, make sure to get professional help. Depression is one of—if not the greatest—risk factor for sexual dysfunction.

For your mental break, plan a movie marathon. You can keep it to just the two of you (if you have a significant other) or invite lots of friends. Next, plan the food. No movie marathon is complete without popcorn and other tasty finger foods. You can take the other person (or whole crowd) and go to the store together beforehand where everyone picks out their own favorite treat or you can supply the bottomless popcorn and tell each friend to bring their favorite treat and enough to share. When you're watching, you can keep to a theme that everyone likes, or let each friend choose their own movie.

CHAPTER 13
HAVING KIDS

MAGGIE'S STORY

It wasn't until I was married that I really started thinking about how T1D would impact pregnancy. That got scary. Is it selfish to want to give birth? Am I setting up my baby for failure because my A1c would not be that of a non-diabetic? How about higher chances of my child developing T1D? After consulting with family members within the medical field and doing research, I was encouraged that with the right support I could do it healthily. Fast forward and here I am just starting my second trimester as a T1D mom-to-be. It has been a roller coaster, but I have gathered a strong support team, which now includes a dietitian and a personal trainer on top of my endo and OB/GYN. This has enabled me to maintain confidence and achieve a lower A1c than ever before. Yes, I am more routine and selective about food choices than before baby. Additionally, I am more aggressive with changing my pump settings and asking for help, but it's working better than I imagined. T1D or not, everyone has stuff going on which we could argue makes them fit or unfit for parenthood. I count all the good I'm doing for my body through exercise, nutrition, and spirituality. Every day of this pregnancy has been a learning experience and I'm embracing wins and failures, learning from them, and moving on. One day at a time.

What to Expect

When I was diagnosed with T1D at the age of four, my pediatrician told my mother I would never be able to have kids of my own. Back in the early 90s we did not have fancy continuous glucose monitors (CGMs), insulin pumps, or even long-acting insulin. We have come a long way with diabetes tech, which makes it much easier for women with T1D to have a healthy pregnancy. More than 25 years after being diagnosed, I do not have diabetes complications, I am in good health, and I have two happy and healthy kids.

Before access to improved treatment and therefore better blood sugar, a pregnant woman with T1D had a much higher risk of spontaneous abortion, stillbirth, giving birth to a baby with heart and kidney defects or a very large weight for gestational age (known as macrosomia). Babies with macrosomia weigh over 8 pounds, 13 ounces at delivery. Macrosomia can cause a difficult and stressful delivery, increase the chances of a Cesarean section, and injure the baby during birth. Babies born with macrosomia are also at a higher risk for obesity and metabolic diseases later in life.

However, by having good diabetes control months before pregnancy and by keeping good control while eating a healthy diet, consistently exercising, and continually adjusting insulin levels throughout pregnancy as needed, most women with T1D can have a safe pregnancy and delivery without birth defects or complications, similar to that of a woman without diabetes.

Because of the better control, a pregnant woman with T1D today only has a very slightly increased risk of stillbirth compared to a mother without diabetes (2 percent versus 1 percent). The ever-so-slight increase is mostly due to a higher rate of serious birth defects that can be reduced with good preconception blood sugar.

Pregnancy is a lot of work without diabetes. When you add diabetes to the mix, some days pregnancy feels like a full-time job. First of all, you'll likely gain more weight than the usual pregnant mom during the first trimester because you will be more sensitive to insulin and also be very cautious to stay in the very strict recommended target blood-sugar ranges. The more tightly controlled you are, coupled with your increased sensitivity to insulin (in the beginning at least), the greater your chance of having lows and your need to be constantly chewing on glucose tabs or some other fast-acting sugar.

With my first pregnancy, I hate to say it, but I purchased a giant bag of Sour Patch Kids to treat my lows and kept it in my desk at work as a dietetic intern. The recommendation for weight gain for the first trimester is 1 to 5 pounds; I gained 13. During that first ultrasound, I was convinced that my baby was, in fact, a giant Sour Patch Kid. In my second trimester, I only gained about half of what the American Pregnancy Association (APA) recommends, then I gained the usual 1 to 2 pounds per week for my last semester. I had the same peculiar weight gain pattern for my second baby, but since it was my second time around, I wasn't concerned. So yes, you'll likely be worried about trying to stick to the recommended weight gain schedule. However, if you instead focus on eating a healthy diet (for the most part), there's no need to stress about the ebbs and flows of your weight gain patterns.

Then, of course, there are the ultra-strict target blood-sugar recommendations. These recommendations are to keep your baby safe and healthy, but an occasional spike or scary drop isn't going to hurt your baby, so don't panic when it happens. It will happen. You may even have an occasional spike that seems overly stubborn to treat. You are at a higher risk for developing ketones, so you may want to monitor these more closely if you are concerned and call your doctor when needed.

You'll also "research" online way too often and scare yourself by reading all the things that can go wrong with a pregnancy and T1D. In reality, these concerns are not related when you properly manage your diabetes, so please, stop researching! It will drive you nuts and stress you out, and you don't need more stress during all of this.

Of course, you'll stress about not eating due to severe nausea, especially early on in your pregnancy. You'll then look online to find that the recommended foods to treat pregnancy-induced nausea are carbs and more carbs (crackers, pretzels, toast, bananas, applesauce). To add to it, you will be terrified of harming your baby by spiking above the intense target blood-sugar recommendations, so you just sit there, constantly playing the "should I eat that or not eat" game. Let's just say, by the end of your pregnancy, you'll be dreaming of swimming in a pool of Oreos, ice cream, popcorn, and any other high-carb food you deemed a "no-no" for a healthy pregnancy.

And there's also the exercise recommendation. Some days you'll feel so low energy that just the thought of walking up and down the stairs for a glass of water counts for you. You'll think that this 150 minutes per week of moderate-intensity exercise recommendation was created solely to make you feel guilty. . . .

To add to it all, expect to become great friends with your obstetrician because you will be spending a lot of time together. With T1D, you may need additional screenings and appointments, but you can expect to see your obstetrician about once a month for the first seven months. Then around 30 to 32 weeks' gestation, you will need to check your baby's heart with non-stress tests two to three times a week until delivery. If your baby is not passing his or her stress test or your baby is measuring greater than what he or she should be based on the week of gestation, your OB/GYN may feel it is better to induce sooner rather than later. However, note that ultrasounds used to estimate a baby's weight can be off by 15 percent or more.

If you have kept your blood sugar in good control, it is reasonable to wait for labor to start on its own. However, waiting beyond 40 weeks is generally not recommended. So, if you don't feel the baby coming anytime soon and the due date is around the corner, call your obstetrician to set a date and time to be induced. Many practitioners routinely induce labor between 38 and 40 weeks in all healthy mothers who have good control of their diabetes (T1D and T2D).

Having diabetes with pregnancy is stressful. Believe me, I've gone through this twice now. But when all is said and done, the time, energy, worry, stress, and effort will be worth it when you are holding that precious and beautiful little baby.

PASSING ON T1D

As a parent, or a potential parent, we naturally want the best for our progeny. We want to give our kids access to good education, a home where they feel safe and loved, and food so they can be properly nourished. We want our kids to develop into good people, who are kind, hardworking, and successful at their craft. Above all else, we want our kids to be healthy and happy. We hope our kids are spared from sickness or chronic conditions out of fear that the child will be kept from achieving their greatest potential and level of happiness. My own experience as well as what I've witnessed with others has shown me that going through difficulties allows people to reach a far greater potential than had they never been challenged at all.

Many parents, or potential parents fear passing T1D to their child. If this is your fear, understand that while there is an increased risk, it is less likely than you'd expect. According to the American Diabetes Association (ADA):

- Children with a father with T1D have a 1 in 17 risk (about 6 percent).

- Children with a mother with T1D have a 1 in 25 risk (4 percent).

- If the T1D mother has her child after she is 25, the risk is reduced to 1 in 100 (1 percent).

- If the parent with T1D was diagnosed with T1D before the age of 11, the risks are doubled.

- If both parents have T1D, the child's risk ranges from 10 to 25 percent.

PRECONCEPTION + PREGNANCY TARGETS

All pregnancies come with risks but having pre-existing T1D before getting pregnant increases the risk of certain complications for you and your baby. However, according to the American Diabetes Association (ADA), you can reduce these risks to nearly that of someone without diabetes by achieving a preconception and pregnancy A1c of 6.5 percent or lower. During pregnancy, less than 6.0 percent is optimal if you can achieve it without significant hypoglycemia. The A1c for someone without diabetes is between 4.0 and 5.6 percent. The closer to normal while avoiding lows, the lower the risk of miscarriage, birth defects, or stillbirth. If the idea of hitting below a 6.0 percent A1c makes your jaw drop, know that due to the increased red blood cell turnover during pregnancy, A1c levels fall lower than your actual blood sugar average. So yes, reaching pregnancy goal A1c takes constant effort, but the increased RBC turnover will give you a little help in achieving targets. If your A1c is quite high (especially above 10 percent) continue effective contraception until you reach a lower A1c. Recommended blood-sugar targets during pregnancy include:

- Before meals, fasting, and bedtime: 60 to 99

- After meals: 100 to 129

- Average daily glucose less than or equal to 110 mg/dL

- Achieve less than 6.0 percent A1c (without significant hypoglycemia)

Let me make this clear again. **These are recommendations only.** Stick to these goals as much as you can, but when you go above and below (and you will), don't panic. These recommendations are the goals, but in no way are they absolutes. Periodic highs and lows out of target are not forever damaging your baby. Do the best you can with the recommendations and when you do experience a high or low, treat it as soon as possible while staying safe, and move on.

INSIDE TYPE 1

Deciding to have kids is emotional and a decision that ultimately must be made by you and your significant other. However, as a mother who has had T1D for many years, my advice to you is to not allow the fear of passing diabetes on to your child keep you from having kids if you desire to be a mother or father. Diabetes can be tough, but treatment will continue to improve until there is a cure and the current odds of not passing on diabetes are in your favor. Also, at some point, you have to stop worrying about what could happen and focus on how to make the most of what you've been given.

Am I a bit trigger happy to test my kids' blood sugar when they seem a tad thirsty? Perhaps. As a mother with T1D, my advice is to not hold your breath for something you can't necessarily change or anticipate.

What to Do

It's important to note that you do not have to have a history of perfect blood sugar to be able to have a healthy pregnancy. I have had diabetes for a long time and have had times when I was "figuring life out" which resulted in periods of ho-hum control. However, when I met my husband-to-be, we made the goal together to get my blood sugar to the normal range of that of someone without diabetes. Today, I continually work on keeping my A1c consistently in the 5s.

I bring this up every time I work with a young woman who feels discouraged because she fears she has already done too much damage to her body to be able to have a healthy pregnancy. If you have had this thought, stop right there.

For the safety of the baby, use contraception if you have an elevated A1c and when you are not wanting to get pregnant. When you are ready, make it a goal to try to hit pregnancy blood-sugar targets, but don't beat yourself up when you have an off day. Work with your doctor closely and hit a 6.5% or below for a minimum of six months before discontinuing your contraception.

Also, if you feel the pre-conception and pregnancy blood-sugar targets are unfathomable, you are not alone. However, I want you to know that through the years, I have met many newly pregnant mothers who haven't always had the greatest control in the past, but there is something that often switches in a mother's brain when she realizes that her blood sugar isn't just affecting herself. Take it day by day, and make sure you have the right medical and support team when you need extra help.

DIABETES + FERTILITY

If you decide that you and your partner are ready to have a baby, the next step is to make sure both of you are preconception ready and given the green light. Many couples, however, deal with infertility and if you have T1D, you may have a higher risk of fertility issues.

T1D, when well controlled, does not cause infertility directly; however, having an autoimmune condition (especially one that is related to hormones) increases your risk of having some other condition that may impact fertility.

There are numerous conditions that can cause infertility in men and women, and the signs and symptoms can vary greatly. For men, signs of infertility issues are often seen as changes in sex drive, testicular pain, and problems with erection or ejaculation. For women, common infertility signs are periods that are irregular, painful, or heavy, or no periods, pain during sex, and symptoms of hormonal issues (weight gain, facial hair, reduced sex drive, thinning hair, dry or flaky skin). If you or your partner have any of these conditions or find anything else out of the ordinary, it is important to let your doctor know so you can be properly assessed and treated.

WHAT TO ASK THE DOCTOR

For men:

1. How does my blood sugar affect fertility?
2. Do any of my current medications affect fertility?
3. What vitamins should I take to increase fertility?

For women:

1. How long do I need to reach my preconception targets before stopping contraception?
2. What are my pregnancy blood-sugar targets?
3. Do I need to check my eyes and kidneys?
4. Do I need to stop any medications before becoming pregnant?
5. What vitamins should I be taking for preconception and pregnancy?
6. Who do I contact after getting a positive pregnancy test?

YOU DO YOU

Deciding to have kids is a life-changing decision and one that shouldn't be taken lightly. This is another very personal decision, but if you are worried about your health and how it could affect a growing baby, there are other options. Perhaps, diabetes aside, you feel that adoption is right for you and your family. I have a patient, who is also a friend, who had two perfectly healthy children naturally, but she and her partner decided that carrying a third child would be too stressful and risky for her health. She was so grateful to her T1D for putting her on this path, because it brought her and her family to this place where they will be welcoming an adopted newborn in the coming months. Sometimes, the very thing that others perceive as a challenge (T1D) can be just the thing to push you to grow and expand in a beautiful way.

Frequently Asked Questions

What type of obstetrician should I use if I have T1D during pregnancy? If you are in good control, you can use an obstetrician who doesn't necessarily specialize in high-risk pregnancies as long as you have an endocrinologist, a CDCES, or a PCP who oversees your insulin management and medical care. If you are more high-risk or need additional medical care, I recommend seeking out a maternal fetal medicine specialist. These are high-risk obstetricians who specialize in managing diabetes in pregnancy. Ask your endo for a recommendation and a referral. As always, check to make sure the specialist is in-network with your insurance before making the visit.

What if I'm already pregnant and my A1c is high? It is important to get in to see your endo ASAP and work closely to figure out how to lower your A1c. An abrupt lowering of A1c can be harmful to your baby and your health, especially if you have proliferative retinopathy. Don't panic, but you will need to work closely with your endo to normalize your blood sugar at a rate that minimizes damage to your and your baby's health.

What if I have high blood sugar while I'm pregnant? This will happen—don't freak out. Just try to safely bring it back down to target ranges as soon as possible. If you are unable to bring it down quickly, troubleshoot if you have expired insulin, a bad site, or ketones. If you have tried a new insulin and it still isn't coming down after about two hours, call your endo clinic or urgent care.

For a break, set aside five minutes to meditate. Meditation can help reduce stress, control anxiety, boost mood, and improve blood sugar. Start by finding a place where you won't be disrupted. Set a timer for five minutes, turn on some healing music, sit in a comfortable position, and close your eyes. When clearing your mind, instead of trying to think of nothing, focus on just "being." Try to visualize the tension leaving your body from your head to your toes, escaping your body with every breath. Don't worry if it is awkward at first, with practice it will become easier.

CHAPTER 14
ALCOHOL

MONICA'S STORY

When I turned 21, I wanted to see what the hype around alcohol was all about. I wasn't a big drinker, but I found the drink called Sex on the Beach. It has orange juice, cranberry juice, vodka, and peach schnapps. I never thought about how much sugar it had it in until I checked my blood sugar because I wasn't feeling so good—not because of the alcohol but because of my diabetes. It turns out I was at 389 and needed to correct.

Now I drink socially but I try to stick with diet sodas and vodka that I don't particularly care for, but such cocktails don't disrupt my blood sugar control as much as others. On a celebration night I will drink my Sex on the Beach or a strawberry daiquiri but, of course, count the carbs. Having diabetes has really changed this whole aspect of my life! I may have to put in more thought before celebrating with friends or at a special occasion, and I may have to be a bit picky about my choices, but after years of close-monitoring my blood sugar during my "drinking experiments," I've gotten pretty good at dosing insulin for when it's worth it.

What to Expect

Excessive drinking is unhealthy for anyone, with or without diabetes. However, this doesn't mean you have to forever commit to a life of abstinence. Research has shown that when consumed in moderation, alcohol may even have heart-protective health benefits. However, the dose makes the poison—with or without diabetes. If someone chooses to drink more than moderately, it can increase complications that affect every organ in their body and increase the risk for certain cancers. While most people are aware of the long-term complications from excessive drinking, the short-term complications can cause just as much, or even more, trouble for someone with diabetes.

The organ most affected in the short- and long term is your liver. You can think of your liver as the blood recycler that tries to get rid of the garbage from what you eat or drink. It protects your body from potentially harmful substances and metabolizes drugs. Another important job of the liver is to regulate blood sugar by packaging the extra energy (glucose) from the food and drink you consume into glycogen (densely compacted glucose). During times of fasting or in between meals, the liver breaks down this glycogen back into glucose so your body can use it for energy. Your liver is constantly in between states of building up and breaking down glycogen stores in order to maintain a stable blood sugar. However, wherever mechanisms relating to blood sugar are involved is where someone with diabetes can get into trouble.

When someone drinks, the liver sees the alcohol as poison and therefore goes into detoxification mode. When your liver switches gears to cleanse the blood, it shifts its focus away from maintaining blood-sugar levels and gives its attention to clearing the body of the "poison." This switch can cause blood glucose levels to drop. A person with a normal functioning pancreas would automatically reduce insulin levels as the available glucose levels decreased. When someone with diabetes drinks, though, it can be rather tricky to match up not only the right amount, but the correct timing of insulin. The more you drink, the harder it is to predict and control your blood sugar. To add to the confusion, consuming sugar in the form of beers, wines, ciders, or perhaps a liquor or spirit in a cocktail with juice, soda, or, say, a margarita mix can cause an initial spike in blood sugar and also make the whole ordeal even more difficult and unpredictable. Before you drink, ask yourself the following questions:

- Is my diabetes in good control?
- Does my health care team agree that I can have alcohol?
- Do I know how alcohol can affect me and my blood sugar?

If you can say yes to all three of these questions, it's likely okay to drink, but make sure to do so cautiously and in moderation. Know how alcohol affects you and understand your own personal limits.

ALCOHOL-RELATED HYPOGLYCEMIA

Alcohol reduces the liver's ability to break down glycogen into glucose which keeps your blood sugar from going too low. Because of this, the more alcohol you drink, the more at risk you are for severe alcohol-induced hypoglycemia.

If someone with T1D doesn't understand the effects of alcohol on blood sugar, they could mistakenly give too much insulin because of the rise in blood sugar from the sugar in a sweetened alcoholic beverage. That person may then go to sleep thinking all is well because they are in the target glucose range, but then wake up in the wee hours of the night drenched in a cold sweat from having a severe low. Left untreated, especially since alcohol decreases coherency, too much alcohol and too much insulin combined can lead to unconsciousness and seizures. This scenario is only intensified when someone drinks excessively to the point of blackout. To top it off, every person reacts differently to alcohol, which can make the timing of a blood sugar drop rather unpredictable. A drop can happen anywhere from immediately after drinking up to 12 hours later, and sometimes can affect insulin sensitivity for up to 24 hours.

It is also important to note that there is a lot of overlap between symptoms of a low and someone who is drunk. Symptoms include drowsiness, slurred speech, and poor coordination.

ALCOHOL-RELATED HYPERGLYCEMIA

On the flip side, you may have experienced blood sugar that shoots up to the 300s after drinking. This may be confusing because we just looked at how drinking lowers blood sugar.

High blood sugar is common because alcoholic drinks contain carbs. Beer is produced by fermented grains. Wine is produced by fermented grapes, and cider is produced by fermented fruits such as apples and pears. Grains, grapes, and fruits all contain carbs. Then you have the hard stuff such as liquor or spirits used in cocktails. Sugary cocktails and mixers can really get you into trouble because they usually contain a variety of different high-sugar syrups, juices, and sodas to create the desired blend and taste.

Bottom line, it is best to drink something that is low-carb such as sparkling water or perhaps even a little diet soda mixed with a squirt of lime or lemon, and gin, whiskey, tequila, or vodka. By going this route, you won't have to guess your exact insulin needs to offset the sugar in the drink. The lower the amount of carbs in the drink, the less insulin you'll require, which leads to a much safer, more predictable 12 to 24 hours after drinking.

When you are first diagnosed, you may have been told that you should completely avoid alcohol from now on because of the detrimental effects on health. This may be fine with some people, but if you are used to having an occasional drink during celebrations, birthday parties, or a spontaneous happy hour with your friends, this information can feel like diabetes has officially ruined your social life. My advice is to have an open dialogue with your doctor about your concerns. During this conversation, tell the truth about how often and how much you actually drink. The more honest you are, the better your doctor can give you advice specific to your situation. If you don't say anything but have every intention to continue to drink, you could get yourself into a really scary predicament. Excessive drinking is harmful for anyone, but by understanding how to drink in moderation and by knowing how alcohol personally affects you, you can drink responsibly, stay safe, and still be able to join in on the celebrations with your workmates, friends, and family.

What to Do

When you want to go out with friends to drink, make sure you have a buddy along who knows how to distinguish drinking behavior from diabetes reaction behavior (such as low-inhibitions versus low blood sugar, and nausea and vomiting from DKA versus intoxication).

Once you've talked to your doctor, and feel that you are pretty well controlled, you can try a drink as an experiment. This can be emotional because having a drink with your friends or for a celebration could have been a way for you to have a good time and let loose. However, diabetes doesn't have to stop you from having a good time. Go out with your friends, stick to a single drink that is low-carb like a lite beer, or a cocktail that uses diet soda. Use this as an experiment. Have your single low-carb drink without insulin but drink it with a meal and take your usual dose for that. This will help you assess how alcohol affects you. To make your drink last, sip slowly, and you are welcome to drink other non-alcoholic beverages that are also low-carb. To help with future situations, you can take a mental (or physical) note of how the alcohol affected you. With time and a little experimenting, you will find the routine that works for you, allows you to still have a good time, but that also keeps you safe.

HOW TO DRINK SAFELY WITH DIABETES

You get it. There are risks and adverse health effects associated with drinking, especially when you have diabetes. However, here are a few tips on how to drink responsibly:

Talk to your doctor: Your doctor can teach you how to modify your insulin to keep you from having crazy highs and scary lows.

Inform your friends: Being drunk and being low can look very similar. Make sure to let the friends who are with you know how to identify a low from acting drunk and what they can do to help you. Also, wearing some sort of diabetes identification bracelet can be useful if you ever become unconscious.

Eat before you go: Always eat something with slow-acting carbs, such as a food that contains fat and protein, before you go out. Doing so can help prevent alcohol-induced low blood sugar and can help your body better process the alcohol consumed.

Know your alcohol: Stick to the low-carb stuff. If you feel confident, you can slowly try others, but if you feel that the low-carb stuff works best, there's no need to change it.

Monitor closely: Make sure to test before, during, and after drinking— before you go to bed, perhaps during the night, and then again when you wake up. Remember, if checking this many times gives you anxiety, consider a CGM.

Increase BG target: It is recommended to treat a blood sugar of 140 or below as a low. If your blood sugar is below 100 after drinking, you will need to use something like glucose tabs in order to bring your blood sugar up quickly. If you are about to go to sleep for the night, and your blood sugar is sitting between 100 and 140, eat a snack that contains a modest amount of carbs and protein such as a slice of wheat toast with peanut butter.

Be ready: Alcohol can do crazy things to your blood sugar, so brace yourself for the unexpected, especially if it's your first time since being diagnosed. Bring your supplies and make sure you have glucose tabs or some sort of fast-acting sugar that can bring your blood sugar up quickly if needed.

WHAT TO ASK THE DOCTOR

1. With my current level of blood-sugar control, can I drink in moderation?
2. How do I adjust my insulin to stay safe while dinking?
3. Where should my blood sugar be before bed after drinking?
4. How do I stay safe with my diabetes if I had a bit more than the recommended amount?
5. If I feel I have a drinking problem, who can I contact for help?

YOU DO YOU

When it comes to alcohol, everybody is different. A glass of wine around 8 p.m. can cause a significant drop in blood sugar a couple of hours later for one person, but no change at all for you. Having diabetes means you will be constantly experimenting with how life impacts your blood sugar. New insulin types, different treatments, foods, and types and amounts of alcohol will all affect your diabetes. Beers, wines, ciders, and cocktails each have different amounts of fermentation, and come from different sources of carbs. Then there are the different brands and mixes within each category. You may find that a bottle of lite beer takes one unit of insulin, while a glass of wine takes two.

Whenever you are trying something that you have never done before (at least since being diagnosed) you need to start small. Starting small is not only better for your health, it makes diabetes a lot easier to work with. Remember, everybody is different, find what works for you and keeps you safe and generally well-controlled.

Frequently Asked Questions

What are long-term effects of excessive drinking? Drinking, especially excessive drinking can damage your heart, liver, brain, pancreas, and really every organ because alcohol is absorbed in the blood and circulates throughout your entire body.

What are the benefits of moderate drinking? The latest guidelines make it clear that no one should begin drinking in hopes for potential health benefits. Avoiding alcohol is best, but if you are a light-to-moderate drinker and are healthy, you can likely continue your ways as long as you do so responsibly. While there is research that shows that light-to-moderate occasional drinking may reduce the risk of dying from heart disease or stroke, even stronger research suggests that eating a healthy diet and regular exercise is much more protective for long-term heart- and overall health.

If wine and a cocktail have the same amount of carbs, do they affect my blood sugar the same? It's important to note that fermented sugar (like from wine or beer) doesn't spike your blood sugar as sharply as a sugary cocktail, even if the carb count is the same. This is due to the fermentation process of the sugar in wines, ciders, and beers compared to the simple sugar in an unfermented juice, syrup, or mixer in a cocktail.

Why can men tolerate more alcohol than women? Scientists have discovered that women produce smaller amounts of alcohol dehydrogenase (ADH), an enzyme released in the liver that breaks down alcohol in the body. Additionally, fat holds onto alcohol, while water helps the body get rid of it faster. The average woman has between 21 and 33 percent body fat while the average man has around 8 to 19 percent body fat. The leaner the individual (lower body fat percentage), the higher the amounts of body water and lean muscle mass. The takeaway: The lower ADH enzyme, higher body fat composition, and the lower muscle mass can be pointed to as the reasons women generally tolerate less alcohol than do men.

JUST ONE THING

My final message for you is to make sure to appreciate every small victory with diabetes—and life in general. You are going to go through ebbs and flows of motivation and ups and downs with your level of diabetes control. That's life. So don't beat yourself up when it happens, and don't be afraid to call out for help when you need a friend. As humans, we all need a lifeline at times. You have many friends, other T1Ds, T1D communities, providers, and educators who understand and want to be there to lessen your burden. Always remember: You are not alone.

Glossary

A1c (hemoglobin A1c or HbA1c): Measure of the average blood glucose level over the past two to three months

Autoimmune disorder: Disorder in which your body's immune system attacks its own tissues

Basal insulin (background insulin): Slow, continuous delivery of insulin to keep blood sugar stable between meals, measured in units per hour

Beta cells: Cells located in the islets of langerhans of the pancreas that make and release insulin

Blood glucose/blood sugar (BG): Level of glucose (sugar) in the blood, measured in mg/dL (milligrams per deciliter)

Bolus: Dose of insulin delivered by a pump to cover food consumed (food bolus) or high blood sugar (correction bolus)

Carb ratio (insulin-to-carbohydrate ratio): Number of grams of carbs covered by 1 unit of insulin

Certified diabetes care and education specialist (CDCES): Healthcare provider who specializes in working with diabetes and has passed a board exam to instruct people in diabetes self-management

Continuous glucose monitor (CGM): Handheld personal device that uses wireless technology to collect blood-sugar readings from a small sensor inserted under the skin

Correction factor (insulin sensitivity factor or ISF): Number of blood glucose (mg/dL) lowered by 1 unit of insulin

Dawn phenomenon: Rise in blood sugar early in the morning due to an increase in hormones

Diabetic ketoacidosis (DKA): This is an emergency condition in which the body has extremely high blood-sugar levels along with a severe lack of insulin, causing the body to break down fat and produce ketones which can be poisonous to the body

Endocrinologist: Board-certified physician who treats issues related to the endocrine system (hormone-related), including diabetes

Fasting blood glucose (FBG): Blood-sugar test after fasting (typically in the morning before food)

Glucagon emergency kit: Kit containing glucagon (hormone used to quickly raise blood glucose), available through syringe or nasal spray to prevent severe hypoglycemia; typically used with T1D who has become unconscious

Glucose: Primary source of energy for the cells derived mostly from carbohydrates from food and drink

Hyperglycemia: High blood sugar or high blood glucose

Hypoglycemia: Low blood sugar, low blood glucose, or insulin reaction

Insulin pump: Small mechanical device that delivers insulin using rapid-acting insulin as basal or bolus

Lipohypertrophy: Built-up scar tissue that occurs when someone overuses an area for syringes or pump sites causing skin to swell and nodes to develop; injected insulin will not be absorbed as well and can cause unpredictable blood sugar

Target range: Ideal range for blood sugar: 80 to 130 before meals; below 180 after meals

Resources

WEBSITES

Ariel Warren, RDN, CD, CDCES blog — arielwarren.com

Affordable Insulin Project — affordableinsulinproject.org

American Diabetes Association — diabetes.org

Beyond Type 1 — Beyondtype1.org

Daily Diabetes Meal Planning Guide — https://www.lillydiabetes
.com/assets/pdf/eldups_pp-ls-us-0165_meal_pln_gd_web_lo_rt4.2
_clean.pdf

Harvard Health Publishing — health.harvard.edu

Joslin Diabetes Center — joslin.org

Juvenile Diabetes Research Foundation — JDRF.org

Take Control of Your Diabetes — tcoyd.org

BOOKS

Bright Spots & Landmines by Adam Brown

Sugar Surfing by Stephen W. Ponder

Think Like a Pancreas by Gary Scheiner

PODCASTS

Diabetes Connections with Stacey Simms

Diabetes Core Update, American Diabetes Association

Juicebox Podcast: Type 1 Diabetes

SUPPORT

Beyond Type 1 — community.beyondtype1.org

Diabetes Daily — diabetesdaily.com/forum

JDRF TypeOneNation — typeonenation.org

American Diabetes Association — community.diabetes.org

References

Affordable Insulin Project (website). Accessed 14 Sept. 2019. http ://affordableinsulinproject.org/.

American Diabetes Association. "Glycemic Targets: Standards of Medical Care in Diabetes—2018." *Diabetes Care* 41, supp. 1 (Jan. 2018): S55-S64. doi: 10.2337 /dc18-S006.

Bădescu, S. V., C. Tătaru, L. Kobylinska, E. L. Georgescu, D. M. Zahiu, A. M. Zăgrean, and L. Zăgrean. "The Association between Diabetes Mellitus and Depression." *Journal of Medicine and Life* 9, no. 2 (Apr.–Jun. 2016): 120–125. https://www.ncbi.nlm.nih.gov/pmc/articles/PMC4863499/.

Barnard, Katharine, Janet James, David Kerr, Peter Adolfsson, Asher Runion, and George Serbedzija. "Impact of Chronic Sleep Disturbance for People Living with T1 Diabetes." *Journal of Diabetes Science and Technology* (1 Dec. 2015). doi: 10.1177/1932296815619181.

Chamberlain, James J., Rita Rastogi Kalyani, Sandra Leal, Andrew S. Rhinehart, Jay H. Shubrook, Neil Skolnik, and William H. Herman. "Treatment of Type 1 Diabetes: Synopsis of the 2017 American Diabetes Association Standards of Medical Care in Diabetes." *Annals of Internal Medicine* 3, no. 167 (3 Oct. 2017): 439–498. doi: 10.7326/M17-1259.

Chetan, M. R., M. H. Charlton, C. Thompson, R. P. Dias, R. C. Andrews, and P. Narendran. "The Type 1 Diabetes 'Honeymoon' Period Is Five Times Longer in Men Who Exercise: A Case–Control Study." *Diabetic Medicine: A Journal of the British Diabetic Association* 36, no. 1 (21 Jun. 2019): 127–128. 10.1111/dme.13802.

"Glycemic Targets: *Standards of Medical Care in Diabetes—2019.*" Diabetes Journals. Accessed 11 December 2019. https://care.diabetesjournals.org /content/42/Supplement_1/S61

Gray, Alison and Rebecca J. Threlkeld. "Nutritional Recommendations for Individuals with Diabetes." *Endotext.* 13 Oct. 2019. https://www.ncbi.nlm.nih.gov /books/NBK279012/.

Karhunen, L. J., K. R. Juvonen, A. Huotari, A. K. Purhonen, and K. H. Herzig. "Effect of Protein, Fat, Carbohydrate and Fibre on Gastrointestinal Peptide Release in Humans." *Regulatory Peptides* 149, nos. 1–3 (Aug. 2008): 70–78. doi:10.1016 /j.regpep.2007.10.008.

Lue, Tom F. "Sexual Dysfunction in Diabetes." *Endotext*. 27 Feb. 2017. https ://www.ncbi.nlm.nih.gov/books/NBK279101/.

Masood, Wajeed and Kalyan R. Uppaluri. "Ketogenic Diet." *StatPearls*. 21 Mar. 2019. https://www.ncbi.nlm.nih.gov/books/NBK499830/.

Mottalib, Adham, Megan Kasetty, Jessica Y Mar, Taha Elseaidy, Sahar Ashrafzadeh, and Osama Hamdy. "Weight Management in Patients with Type 1 Diabetes and Obesity." *Current Diabetes Reports* 17, no. 10 (23 Aug. 2017): 92. doi: 1007/s11892-017-0918-8.

Mul, Joram D., Kristin I. Stanford, Michael F. Hirshman, and Laurie J. Goodyear. "Exercise and Regulation of Carbohydrate Metabolism." *Progress in Molecular Biology and Translational Science* 135 (2015): 17–37. doi: 10.1016/bs.pmbts .2015.07.020.

Paterson, Megan A., Kirstine J. Bell, Susan M. O'Connell, Carmel E. Smart, Amir Shafat, and Bruce R. King. "The Role of Dietary Protein and Fat in Glycaemic Control in Type 1 Diabetes: Implications for Intensive Diabetes Management." *Current Diabetes Reports*. (2015). doi: 10.1007/x11892-015-0630-5.

"Saving Money on Health Insurance: Income Levels & Savings." HealthCare.gov. Accessed 13 Oct. 2019. https://www.healthcare.gov/lower-costs/qualifying-for -lower-costs/.

"TrialNet Announces Type 1 Diabetes Prevention Advancement." Type 1 Diabetes TrialNet. Accessed 19 Sept. 2019. https://www.trialnet.org/.

Trief, Paula M., Yawen Jiang, Roy Beck, Peter J. Huckfeldt, Tara Knight, Kellee M. Miller, and Ruth S. Weinstock. "Adults with Type 1 Diabetes: Partner Relationships and Outcomes. *Journal of Health Psychology* (2015). doi: 10.1177/1359105315605654.

"TSA Travel Tips: Travelers with Diabetes or Other Medical Conditions." (blog). Transportation Security Administration. 1 Apr. 2014. https://www.tsa.gov/blog /2014/04/01/tsa-travel-tips-travelers-diabetes-or-other-medical-conditions.

"Types of Insulin." HealthLinkBC. Updated 25 Jul. 2018. https://www.healthlinkbc .ca/health-topics/aa122570.

Umpierrez, Guillermo E., and David C. Klonoff. "Diabetes Technology Update: Use of Insulin Pumps and Continuous Glucose Monitoring in the Hospital." *Diabetes Care* 41, no. 8 (Aug. 2018): 1579–1589. doi: 10.2337/dci18-0002.

von Frankenberg, Anize D., Anna Marina, Xiaoling Song, Holly S. Callahan, Mario Kratz, and Kristina M. Utzschneider. "A High-Fat, High-Saturated Fat Diet Decreases Insulin Sensitivity without Changing Intra-Abdominal Fat in Weight -Stable Overweight and Obese Adults." *Diabetology & Metabolic Syndrome* 7, suppl. 1 (Nov. 2015). doi: 10.1186/1758-5996-7-S1-A234.

White, Nicole D. "Alcohol Use in Young Adults with Type 1 Diabetes Mellitus." *American Journal of Lifestyle Medicine* (26 Jul. 2017). doi: 10.1177/1559827617722137.

Index

screening for, 13–14
symptoms, 4–5
typical day in the life with, 23–25
Type 2 diabetes (T2D), 4

U

Ultra long-acting insulin, 20

W

Weight gain, 27–28, 46, 117–119
Weight loss, 116–117, 119–122
Work life, 86–88

Acknowledgments

To my best friend and husband, Jace: for always believing that I could do better and work harder, while also always loving me for who I am.

To my beautiful children, Barrett and Zona: for simply being my babies. I cherish you with all my heart. You motivate me to live well with diabetes every day.

To my parents, Mark and Carol: for raising me, loving me, and always being wonderful examples of what parents can be for a child.

To my in-laws, Scott and Kelly: for always treating me as your own and for being such admirable people whom I love and sincerely appreciate.